POCKET GUIDE TO
SPIROMETRY

3E

The third edition of this guide is dedicated to the memory of Rob Pierce.

3E

POCKET GUIDE TO

Spirometry

David P. Johns
PhD, CRFS, FANZSRS
Primary Research Fellow, Menzies Research Institute
University of Tasmania

Rob Pierce
MBBS, MD, FRACP, FCCP
Former Professor/Director of Respiratory and Sleep Medicine
University of Melbourne and Austin Hospital

Mc
Graw
Hill
Education

NOTICE
Medicine is an ever-changing science. As new research and clinical experience broaden our knowledge, changes in treatment and drug therapy are required. The editors and the publisher of this work have checked with sources believed to be reliable in their efforts to provide information that is complete and generally in accord with the standards accepted at the time of publication. However, in view of the possibility of human error or changes in medical sciences, neither the editors, nor the publisher, nor any other party who has been involved in the preparation or publication of this work warrants that the information contained herein is in every respect accurate or complete. Readers are encouraged to confirm the information contained herein with other sources. For example, and in particular, readers are advised to check the product information sheet included in the package of each drug they plan to administer to be certain that the information contained in this book is accurate and that changes have not been made in the recommended dose or in the contraindications for administration. This recommendation is of particular importance in connection with new or infrequently used drugs.

Reprinted 2018
First published 2003; Second edition 2007; Third edition 2011

Copyright © 2011 David Johns and Rob Peirce
Illustrations and design Copyright ©McGraw-Hill Australia Pty Limited
Additional owners of copyright are acknowledged in on-page credits and on the acknowledgments page.

Every effort has been made to trace and acknowledge copyrighted material. The authors and publishers tender their apologies should any infringement have occurred.

National Library of Australia Cataloguing-in-Publication Data

Author:	Johns, David Peter, 1952-
Title:	Pocket guide to spirometry / David P. Johns and Rob Pierce.
Edition:	3rd ed.
ISBN:	9780071016193 (pbk.)
Notes:	Includes index.
Subjects:	Spirometry—Handbooks, manuals, etc.Pulmonary function tests—Handbooks, manuals, etc.

Other Authors/ Contributors:	Pierce, Rob, 1947-2009
Dewey Number:	616.24075

Published in Australia by
McGraw-Hill Education (Australia) Pty Ltd
Level 33, 680 George Street, Sydney NSW 2000
Acquisitions editor: Fiona Richardson
Art director: Astred Hicks
Cover design: Patricia McCallum and Astred Hicks
Internal design: Patricia McCallum
Production editor: Natalie Crouch
Copyeditor: Nicole McKenzie
Proofreader: Annabel Adair
Indexer: Glenda Browne
Typeset in Palatino 8.5/10.5pt by Midland Typesetters, Australia
Printed in Australia by Griffin Digital

THIRD EDITION

This is the best book for learning how to perform and interpret spirometry in primary care settings. Using a spirometer is like driving a car: even teenagers can quickly learn, but it takes several weeks of guidance from an expert, followed by years of experience to do it well. This book, written for the beginner, provides practical guidance from world-class experts. Take it home and read it in a comfortable chair, then keep it next to your spirometer as a reference. The operators' manual for your spirometer just tells you what buttons to press, but not how to get good quality results or how to interpret the numbers and graphs. The spirometry guidelines from professional organizations (like those published by the American Thoracic Society and the European Respiratory Society in 2005) contain too much detail and referenced rationale for someone who wants to learn the basics.

Spirometry is greatly underutilized for pediatric patients with asthma-like symptoms and to follow treatment responses. Spirometry is also underutilized for detecting COPD in the 20% of smokers over age 40 who have slowly developed the disease. A daily inhaler for COPD must not be prescribed without using a spirometer to confirm the O in COPD, since many adult smokers have a chronic cough or dyspnea which is not due to COPD.

Several strenuous, athletic-like breathing maneuvers are needed to accurately measure the FEV_1 and FVC. Very few other medical tests require patient cooperation and effort. This book tells you how to demonstrate these maneuvers and recognize when the inhalation or exhalation efforts were inadequate, leading to falsely low values which often cause incorrect interpretations. You really should buy this easy-to-read spirometry guide.

Paul Enright, MD, Professor of Medicine,
The University of Arizona, USA

May 2011

FOREWORD TO THE SECOND EDITION

The second edition of the *Pocket Guide to Spirometry* by David Johns and Rob Pierce is likely to be even more popular than the first as the changes that have been incorporated enhance and update this excellent resource. Additions include incorporation throughout of the 2005 American Thoracic Society and European Respiratory Society joint recommendations on spirometry measurement and interpretation, as well as a change to the more recent and robust reference equations for normal spirometry of Hankinson, Odencrantz and Fedan (1999). Importantly, the succinct and conversational style that has made the book accessible to the full range of health professional readers and the vital sections explaining the underlying physiology of the mechanics of breathing, vital to understanding what is being measured by spirometry, are retained.

This book is useful for all with an interest in optimal measurement and interpretation of spirometry, whether they are novices or are using it as a resource as they acquire further experience. A primary aim of the Australian and New Zealand Society of Respiratory Science is to support and encourage education and training in respiratory science and excellence in respiratory measurement, and it is for this reason that we proudly endorse this excellent publication.

Debbie Burton, New South Wales Representative/Board member,
Australian & New Zealand Society of Respiratory Science

Graham Hall, President,
Australian & New Zealand Society of Respiratory Science

March 2007

FOREWORD TO THE FIRST EDITION

Spirometry is spirometry is spirometry. It matters not if this measurement of lung function is performed in an accredited lung function laboratory at a major hospital, by an occupational health nurse at a remote mining site or by a general physician at his/her practice. The same general principles must apply to all in order to achieve an accurate result. Unfortunately this is not always the case. There is a perception that by simply combining a patient with a spirometer, accurate results of high quality are automatically produced, with apparently little thought afforded to the accuracy of the device performing the measurement, the effort of the subject undertaking the test or the competence of the person supervising the test. Despite the ready availability of internationally accepted guidelines for the performance of spirometry, the literature abounds with reports of spirometry measurements of such poor quality to render it useless at best, to downright dangerous should this result be incorrectly interpreted.

It is now recognised that only a good understanding of lung physiology plus appropriate education in all aspects of spirometry can overcome the problems associated with this measurement. Careful reading of this book will certainly provide readers with a thorough understanding of spirometry from calibration through to interpretation.

This excellent publication, and indeed its precursor—*Spirometry: The Measurement and Interpretation of Ventilatory Function in Clinical Practice*—represents another chapter in the ongoing commitment of David and Rob to raise the standard of spirometry performed in Australia and New Zealand. In this publication, David and Rob have added sections that will be particularly useful at the 'coalface' (e.g. spirometry in children, the FEV_6 and case histories). They have also taken the extra step of including a section on the mechanics of breathing which succinctly demonstrates how normal (and abnormal) physiology can affect measurements of spirometry and greatly assist in its interpretation.

We have no doubt this publication will shortly become the popular spirometry reference book in Australia and New Zealand and strongly endorse its use by all healthcare professionals performing spirometry and indeed all measurements of ventilatory function.

Brenton Eckert, President,
Australian & New Zealand Society of Respiratory Science

Richard Ruffin, President,
Thoracic Society of Australia and New Zealand.

March 2003

CONTENTS

Foreword to the third editon   v
Foreword to the second editon   vi
Foreword to the first editon   vii
Preface   xii
Acknowledgments   xiii
About the authors   xv
Introduction   xvii

Chapter 1   What is spirometry and what are its uses?   1
The function of the lung and lung function tests   1
Indications for spirometry   3
Complications and contraindications   4
Summary   5

Chapter 2   Measurement of ventilatory function   6
The spirogram   6
Indices based on 6-second forced expiration   7
Inspiratory capacity   10
The flow-volume curve or loop   10
Summary   12

Chapter 3   Measurement devices   13
Volume-displacement spirometers   14
Flow spirometers   14
Monitoring devices and peak flow meters   16
Calibration and quality control   17
Factors to consider when choosing a spirometer   21
Summary   22

Chapter 4   How to do spirometry and the
            common problems   23
How to do spirometry   23
Measurements in young children   26
Acceptability and repeatability criteria   26

Back-extrapolation 28
Patient-related problems 30
Instrument-related problems 34
Performing spirometry in the busy clinical practice 34
Summary 35

Chapter 5   Infection control 36
Cross-infection and lung function testing 36
Reducing the risk of cross-infection 37
Summary 38

Chapter 6   Predicted normal values 39
Normal values 39
Summary 41

Chapter 7   Interpretation of spirometry 44
Significant change in spirometry with time 44
Classifying abnormal ventilatory function 45
Grading severity of a ventilatory defect 53
Measuring reversibility of airflow obstruction 54
Airway provocation testing 55
Peak flow monitoring 57
Choosing the appropriate test 59
Summary 60

Chapter 8   Case histories 61
Case 1 62
Case 2 64
Case 3 66
Case 4 68
Case 5 70
Case 6 72
Case 7 74
Case 8 76
Case 9 78
Case 10 80
Case 11 82
Summary 83

Chapter 9   Mechanics of breathing 84
Gas flow through the airways—how airflow is produced 84
Patterns of airflow in the human airways 85
The phenomenon of maximal airflow limitation 87

Theories of airflow obstruction 90
How pulmonary disease affects airflow 93
Summary 94

Chapter 10   Summary 95

Appendix A Equipment standards and validation
            procedures 96
Appendix B Correction of volume and flow to BTPS 99
Appendix C Predicted normal values 102
Glossary 129
References 134
Useful websites 137
Index 138

This third edition of *Pocket Guide to Spirometry* has been updated throughout to comply with the latest spirometry standards developed jointly by the American Thoracic Society and the European Respiratory Society. Predicted normal value tables for FEV_1, FVC, FEV_1/FVC and $FEF_{25-75\%}$ have been completely revised to adhere to Stanojevic et al. (2009) and now seamlessly cover the age range of 4 to 80 years. A number of relatively minor changes and additions have been made to the text and figures, some in response to suggestions by readers, for which we are very grateful. For example, FEV_1/FVC is now expressed throughout as a fraction rather than a percentage and a new case has been added.

Over recent years there has been a growing recognition of the value of spirometry in clinical medicine and physicians are now being encouraged to include the measurement in their clinical practice. However, it is often not appreciated that clinically useful results are critically dependent on the accuracy of the spirometer and the competence of the operator in instructing and motivating the patient to perform the correct breathing manoeuvre.

The main reason for writing this book was to help improve the quality of spirometry measurements and their interpretation, and to encourage the use of spirometry in clinical medicine. We have attempted to provide a practical guide for those involved in the performance and interpretation of spirometry—medical practitioners and assisting nursing staff, respiratory scientists, technologists, technicians, physiotherapists and other healthcare workers.

This book is not intended to be an exhaustive review but rather a guide to help improve the knowledge and techniques of those already doing and interpreting spirometry, and to introduce spirometry to those learning how to do it for the first time. The important facts about the physiology of normal airflow and the pathophysiology underlying spirometric deficits are given, as is practical information about types of spirometers and how the test is actually performed and interpreted. Some common pitfalls and problems are covered in the main text. Case histories taken from clinical practice are used to illustrate the diagnostic value of airflow and lung volume measurement.

In February 2009, Rob Pierce, my co-author on the previous editions of this guide, perished in the raging fires that swept mercilessly through parts of Victoria. Rob's knowledge and enthusiasm for respiratory and sleep medicine, his deep understanding of physiology and his gentle collegiate and supportive nature makes it especially difficult to accept that he is no longer with us, but I am very grateful to have had the privilege to have known and worked with him. Rob and I first met in the mid 1970s at the Brompton Heart and Chest Hospital in the United Kingdom. We have worked together on several educational projects. These include the National Asthma Council (NAC) 'blue' book (*Spirometry: The Measurement and Interpretation of Ventilatory Function in Clinical Practice*); two multimedia CD-ROMs on spirometry; a NAC online book (*Spirometry: The Measurement and Interpretation of Ventilatory Function in Clinical Practice*); and the first and second editions of this guide.

ACKNOWLEDGMENTS

With regard to the last two editions of this book, Rob and I are most grateful to the National Asthma Council who in 1995 published our original handbook on which this book is based (*Spirometry: The Measurement and Interpretation of Ventilatory Function in Clinical Practice*). We are also indebted to two outstanding teachers of respiratory physiology, Dr Alistair Campbell and Professor David Denison. We wish to thank the many colleagues who offered advice and support, especially Professor E. Haydn Walters, Brenton Eckert, Kevin Gain, Debbie Burton, Maureen Swanney, Andrew Coates, Eleonora Side, Sandra Anderson and Peter Rochford. There are also a number of professional organisations to whom we are most grateful for providing valuable advice that has helped maintain the relevance of this book as a practical guide: the Australian and New Zealand Society of Respiratory Science and the Thoracic Society of Australia and New Zealand and Royal College of General Practitioners. Finally, Lesley Pocock, Director of Mediworld Inc., has been extremely helpful in providing professional advice and for the publication of our interactive multimedia CD-ROM on spirometry (*Spirometry*), which includes an abridged electronic version of this book.

In producing the third edition, I am very grateful to Associate Professor Debbie Burton, Dr Jeff Pretto, Professor Paul Enright, Yu Guang Zhang and Gary Noland for reviewing the second edition and providing valuable and constructive feedback. I am also very grateful to Dr Sanja Stanojevic who kindly provided the data for the 'all-age' predicted normal reference tables given in Appendix C. I am also grateful to the publisher, McGraw-Hill Australia, for their encouragement and enthusiasm in producing this edition.

It is most unfortunate that my friend and co-author, Rob Pierce, is no longer with us; however, his spirit and drive remain very much alive and remain an inspiration for this edition.

David P. Johns

David Johns is a respiratory physiologist with a particular interest in research and undergraduate and postgraduate teaching. He is currently Primary Research Fellow at the Menzies Research Institute, Tasmania. He commenced his respiratory career in 1972 at the Brompton Heart and Chest Hospital, United Kingdom, and moved to Australia in 1978 where for the next 23 years he developed and managed respiratory laboratories at Victoria's Austin and Alfred Hospitals. In 2001 David moved to the University of Tasmania to pursue his research and teaching interests. In 2007 he moved to Queensland.

His research interests are focused on the physiological consequences of airway modelling, mathematical modelling of gas exchange, and the development and interpretation of lung function tests. He is actively engaged with the medical profession, national professional organisations, government and industry. He is a principal author of the popular national GP spirometry training course run by the National Asthma Council (NAC).

David has published original research papers, textbooks, online books, book chapters and interactive multimedia CD-ROMs. His contributions to respiratory research were recognised in 2002 when he was awarded Fellowship of the Australian and New Zealand Society of Respiratory Science and received the ANZSRS Research Medal for his contributions to respiratory science.

Rob Pierce

Up until his death in the Victorian Black Saturday fires, Rob Pierce was Professor/Director of Respiratory and Sleep Medicine at the University of Melbourne and the Austin Hospital in Heidelberg, Victoria. He was also a foundation Medical Director of the Institute for Breathing and Sleep (at the Austin), which continues to promote research, education and public advocacy in respiratory and sleep health. Since the early 1980s, he had a long-term association with the respiratory laboratory at the Austin Hospital and led the working group on guidelines for lung function testing for the Thoracic Society of Australia and New Zealand.

His MD thesis was concerned with measurement of lung and lobar volumes and the accuracy of various measurement techniques and was completed at the Brompton Hospital in the United Kingdom. He published extensively in peer-reviewed scientific journals and co-authored with David Johns the interactive CD-ROM, *Spirometry*.

Rob taught respiratory physiology and medicine at University of Melbourne for many years. His clinical research interests included the physiology, function and disease of both lower and upper airways. He was a foundation investigator in the Australasian Sleep Trials Network, which, among other clinical areas, supports research into the impact of sleep on airway physiology and the clinical consequences of sleep-disordered breathing.

INTRODUCTION

[Spirometry] should be readily available and routinely used in medical offices and hospitals where patients with heart and lung diseases are treated.[1]

A great deal can be learned about the mechanical properties of the lungs from measurements of maximal expiration and inspiration. Since Hutchinson first developed the spirometer in 1846, measurements of the so-called dynamic lung volumes and of maximal flows have been used in the detection and quantification of diseases affecting the respiratory system. Over the years it has become obvious that the spirometer and peak flow meter used to measure ventilatory function are as deserving of a place in the family practitioner's surgery as the sphygmomanometer. After all, who would dream of managing hypertension without measurement of blood pressure?

Respiratory disease is a major clinical problem. At the date of publication of this book, about one in nine children and one in 10 adults in some countries, including Australia and New Zealand, have asthma and there is evidence that the prevalence is increasing. In Australia alone over 2.2 million people have a diagnosis of asthma and it is estimated that the health costs associated with the care of people with asthma is as high as $693 million per year. In addition, 10% to 20% of adults over 40 years of age have chronic obstructive pulmonary disease (COPD) with the odds ratio for developing COPD increasing dramatically with smoking and age. Despite these disturbing statistics only 25% to 33% of those with measurable airflow obstruction in general practice have a diagnosis or are aware of their respiratory problem. By the year 2020, COPD will be the third most common overall cause of death, representing 11% of deaths from any cause. In these diseases, spirometry is essential for the diagnosis and the assessment of response to therapy.

---

1. Dr Robert O. Crapo, 'Pulmonary function testing', *New England Journal of Medicine*, 1994, 331(1), pp. 25–30.

There are now simple, accurate, robust and reliable spirometers that enable ventilatory function to be measured in a doctor's surgery as readily as in a hospital respiratory function laboratory. There are also portable devices that enable patients with lung disease to monitor their own progress and the status of their lung disease. The self-monitoring of peak flow by people with asthma and its use to regulate their treatment with anti-inflammatory and bronchodilator drugs is a natural extension of the ease with which ventilatory function can now be monitored reliably.

The role of spirometry in case finding in general practice and in screening of high-risk populations has recently begun to be evaluated in relation to the high prevalence and vast under-diagnosis of respiratory disease in the general population and the even greater prevalence in high-risk populations, for example, smokers over 40 years of age and in certain occupational settings.

It is important to appreciate that the clinical value of spirometric measurements is critically dependent on the correct operation and accuracy of the spirometer, performance of the correct breathing manoeuvre, selection of the best results and use of relevant predicted normal values.

It is very clear, therefore, that spirometry should be readily available in general practice and the measurement of ventilatory capacity should be regarded as mandatory for many patients.

Spirometry training

It is important that staff performing spirometry first attend a comprehensive training course. This is because inadequate training will result in poor quality spirometry that is of little clinical value. As a minimum these courses should provide adequate training in how to:

- maintain and validate the spirometer
- perform the correct breathing manoeuvre
- identify and overcome poor technique
- select and report the results of spirometry.

Lists of spirometry training courses in Australia and New Zealand are available on the websites of the Australian and New Zealand Society of Respiratory Science (www.anzsrs.org.au) and the Thoracic Society of Australia and New Zealand (www.thoracic.org.au).

1

WHAT IS SPIROMETRY AND WHAT ARE ITS USES?

Spirometry is a physiological test of lung function, so in order to introduce it a brief summary of the function of the pulmonary system is appropriate.

THE FUNCTION OF THE LUNG AND LUNG FUNCTION TESTS

The primary function of the lungs is to arterialise mixed venous blood to meet the metabolic demands of the body (Figure 1.1). If the lungs are functioning normally, they will produce arterialised blood of normal composition and they will do this even during strenuous exercise. The lung achieves this by bringing almost the entire output from the heart into intimate contact with the air we breathe. If lung function is normal, at sea level arterial blood will have a P_{CO_2} of about 40 mmHg, a P_{O_2} close to 100 mmHg and an oxygen saturation (S_{O_2}) of about 97%. The lungs have a large reserve and S_{O_2} (often measured non-invasively using a pulse oximeter) at rest remains well preserved until severe lung disease.

Several component processes interact to determine the effectiveness of lung function to meet the metabolic demands of the body's tissues:

- *ventilation*: capacity of the respiratory system to move air into and out of all the gas-exchanging regions of the lung containing pulmonary capillary blood

ventilation

mixed
venous
blood

P_{CO_2} = 46 mmHg
P_{O_2} = 40 mmHg
S_{O_2} = 75%

arterial
blood

P_{CO_2} = 40 mmHg
P_{O_2} = 100 mmHg
S_{O_2} = 97%

perfusion

The lungs arterialise venous blood

Figure 1.1 Simplified model of the lung showing ventilation and blood flow. The average normal adult lung has a total lung capacity of about 6.5 litres, about 300 million alveoli and is almost continuously perfused by a flow of blood equal to the cardiac output. At rest we breathe 5–10 L/min and cardiac output is about 5 L/min. The blood perfusing the alveoli is so thinly spread that at any instant the volume participating in gas exchange is only about 80 mL.

- *pulmonary blood flow*: capacity of the circulatory system to deliver mixed venous blood to all the gas-exchanging regions of the lung
- *diffusion*: passive movement of CO_2 and O_2 across the alveolar–capillary membrane that separates air in the alveoli from blood perfusing the pulmonary capillaries. The process of gas diffusion and pulmonary blood flow are collectively described as the gas-exchange function of the lungs
- *control of ventilation*: regulation of ventilation to ensure adequate arterialisation of mixed venous blood to meet metabolic demands.

Each of these components interacts with the others and all are essential for normal lung function. There is no single test of lung function that will assess all of the above components of lung function, but many tests, each of which will assess one or more of the various components of function. For example:

- Spirometry is the measurement of respired or dynamic lung volumes and assesses ventilatory capacity. It is often measured before and after (i) the administration of bronchodilator agent(s) to assess reversibility, (ii) exercise to assess exercise-induced bronchocon-striction, or (iii) inhalation of an agent that may reduce bronchospasm (e.g. mannitol, methacholine) to quantify airway reactivity.

- Lung volumes assess lung size and represent the structural and physiological limits of the respiratory system.
- Diffusing capacity (or transfer factor) assesses the perfused surface area, thickness and integrity of the alveolar–capillary membrane.
- Arterial blood gas tensions, used in conjunction with the alveolar gas equation, are used to assess gas exchange.
- Exercise tests are used to evaluate the capacity and integrated pulmonary and cardiopulmonary function under conditions of increased metabolic demand.

Although lung function tests are rarely diagnostic by themselves, they can provide valuable clues about the mechanisms underlying the pathophysiological disease process. The clues to be gained depend on a sound understanding of the physiological basis of the measurement, test variability, comparison with normal reference values, and knowledge of how lung disease alters the structure and function of the lungs.

The single most broadly useful non-invasive test of ventilatory lung function is spirometry. This is because impaired ventilatory function, particularly airflow obstruction, is the most common physiological abnormality affecting the lung (e.g. asthma and COPD, chronic obstructive pulmonary disease). The most common cause of impaired ventilatory function is airway narrowing. This may be due to loss of traction from the surrounding lung tissue as in emphysema; inflammation of the walls of the airway, mucus plugging and bronchospasm as in asthma; or to obstruction of the airway lumen caused, for instance, by a tumour. Other causes of impaired ventilatory function include respiratory muscle weakness or paralysis, cardiac enlargement, or alterations to the lung, chest wall or pleura that limit the full expansion or the rate of emptying of the lung.

Spirometry is therefore an important test to detect, quantify and monitor diseases that limit ventilatory capacity—the mechanical properties of the lung and chest wall that affect the lung's volume and the calibre of the airways.

INDICATIONS FOR SPIROMETRY

The following list summarises the wide range of indications for spirometry (see also Miller et al. 2005b):

- detecting and assessing respiratory disease in patients presenting with symptoms of breathlessness either at rest or on exertion, wheeze, cough, stridor, phlegm production, etc.

- assessing respiratory function in all smokers and people exposed to polluted environments and in those with a family history of respiratory disease
- differentiating respiratory from cardiac disease as the cause of breathlessness
- screening for respiratory disease in certain high-risk situations and populations, for example, smokers (especially over 40 years of age), pre-employment in industries in which occupational asthma is prevalent and identifying those at risk from activities such as scuba diving
- diagnosing respiratory disease, differentiating obstructive versus restrictive ventilatory defects, and identifying upper airway obstruction and diseases associated with weakness of the respiratory muscles
- assessing the severity and following the natural history and progression of respiratory and sometimes systemic and neuromuscular diseases
- assessing response to treatment
- assessing impairment from respiratory disease in the workplace and in the settings of pulmonary rehabilitation and compensation for occupational lung disease
- assessing preoperative risk prior to anaesthesia and abdominal or thoracic surgery.

COMPLICATIONS AND CONTRAINDICATIONS

Spirometry is generally a safe, non-invasive procedure. However, it does require maximal effort and subject cooperation, which may result in transient breathlessness, oxygen desaturation, syncope, chest pain and cough. The forced manoeuvre can also induce bronchospasm in patients with poorly controlled asthma. There are a number of clinical circumstances in which the generation of a high positive intra-thoracic pressure and its transmission to vascular, abdominal and other body compartments may be detrimental and thus spirometry is best avoided. The measurement of spirometry is thus normally delayed following:

- recent eye surgery
- recent thoracic and abdominal surgery
- aneurysms (e.g. cerebral, abdominal)
- unstable cardiac function
- haemoptysis of unknown cause (i.e. infection risk)

- pneumothorax
- chest and abdominal pain
- nausea and diarrhoea.

SUMMARY

Spirometry is a very useful non-invasive test to detect, quantify and monitor diseases that limit ventilatory function. The test is relatively easy to perform, although it does require maximal effort and patient cooperation is essential. Spirometry is generally a safe test, although it can induce bronchospasm in patients with poorly controlled asthma and there are several contraindications where it is unwise to proceed with the test.

1

CHAPTER 2

MEASUREMENT OF VENTILATORY FUNCTION

Conventionally, a spirometer is a device used to measure timed expired and inspired volumes, and from these we can calculate how effectively and how quickly the lungs can be emptied and filled. Spirometry is usually recorded as either a *spirogram* (a plot of volume versus time) or *flow-volume curve* or *loop* (a plot of volume versus flow).

THE SPIROGRAM

Figure 2.1 shows two commonly recorded spirograms. The measurements that are usually made are as follows:

- **FVC** (forced vital capacity) and **VC** (vital capacity) are the maximum volume of air that can be expired or inspired during either a forced (FVC) or a slow (VC) manoeuvre. The FVC is normally equal to the VC unless airway closure occurs during the forced expiratory manoeuvre, in which case the VC is higher than FVC. The difference between VC and FVC is often referred to as 'trapped gas'.
- **FEV_1** (forced expired volume in 1 second) is the volume expired in the first second of maximal expiration (initiated after a maximal inspiration) and is a very widely used measure of how quickly full lungs can be emptied.
- **FEV_1/FVC ratio** (or FEV_1/VC) is the FEV_1 expressed as a fraction (or percentage) of the FVC (or VC) (whichever volume is larger) and gives a clinically useful index of airflow limitation. It is essentially

the proportion of the lung volume that can be expired in 1 second and is also referred to as the forced expiratory ratio, FER.

- **$FEF_{25-75\%}$** (forced expiratory flow over the middle half of the FVC manoeuvre) is the average expired flow over the middle half of the FVC manoeuvre and is regarded as a more sensitive measure of peripheral or small airways narrowing than FEV_1. Unfortunately, $FEF_{25-75\%}$ has a wide range of normality, is less reproducible than FEV_1 and is difficult to interpret if the FVC is reduced or increased. (This index was formerly termed the maximal mid-expiratory flow rate, MMEFR.)
- **FET** (forced expiratory time) is the time required to perform the FVC manoeuvre (usually less than 5–6 seconds in adults and 2–3 seconds in children). The FET is increased in the presence of airflow limitation (often > 12 seconds).

INDICES BASED ON 6-SECOND FORCED EXPIRATION

Spirometric indices calculated using a 6-second volume base instead of the FVC are gaining popularity (Ferguson et al. 2000). Stopping the expiratory manoeuvre after 6 seconds has the advantage of decreasing the physical demands of performing spirometry and potentially reducing their coefficient of variation. This is an advantage for patients with significant airway obstruction as well as the elderly and physically impaired. In addition, the variations in FVC due to variations in expiratory time are eliminated if we substitute FVC_6 for FVC. The diagnostic criteria are equivalent to the traditional FVC-based parameters. Many portable spirometers now have these 6-second parameters available in their software.

- **FVC_6** is the largest forced expiratory volume measured during the first 6 seconds. This is similar to FEV_6, which is the forced expiratory volume measure *at* 6 seconds.
- **FEV_1/FVC_6** is FEV_1 expressed as a fraction of the FVC_6.
- **$FEF_{25-75\%6}$** is the forced expiratory flow over the middle half of the FVC_6 manoeuvre.

It is important to use appropriate reference values (i.e. based on a 6-second expiration) when interpreting these indices.

Studies have reported that these parameters are equivalent to the traditional FVC and FEV_1/FVC for the diagnosis of obstructive and restrictive patterns and for predicting decline in smokers (Swanney et al. 2000; Enright, Connett & Bailey 2002). The clinical utility of $FEF_{25-75\%}$ is limited because of the large variation in this index, which

Figure 2.1 Normal spirogram showing the measurements of forced vital capacity (FVC), forced expired volume in one second (FEV_1), forced expiratory flow over the middle half of the FVC ($FEF_{25-75\%}$) and the forced expiratory time (FET). The top panel is a typical recording from a water-sealed (or rolling seal) spirometer with expired volume downward; the bottom panel is a typical spirogram from a dry wedge-bellows spirometer with expired volume upward.

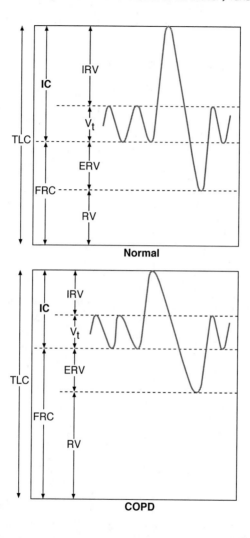

Figure 2.2   The lung volumes and capacities in normal and hyperinflated lungs (e.g. COPD). The inspiratory capacity (IC) is the volume that can be inspired from the functional residual capacity (FRC). TLC = total lung capacity; RV = residual volume; ERV = expiratory reserve volume; IRV = inspiratory reserve volume; V_t = tidal volume.

is partly due to its dependence on FVC. However, using FVC_6 as the volume base may reduce this variation.

INSPIRATORY CAPACITY

The inspiratory capacity (IC) is the maximum volume of air that can be inspired from the end of quiet expiration (from functional residual capacity, FRC, to total lung capacity, TLC)—see Figure 2.2. This index is gaining popularity as a measure of dynamic hyperinflation during exercise and as a measure of the degree of reduced hyper-inflation following the administration of a bronchodilator, especially in COPD (see p. 53).

This measurement of IC using open-circuit spirometry (see Chapter 4) involves switching the patient into this circuit at the end of quiet expiration (i.e. at FRC) and measuring the maximum volume that can be inspired (i.e. to total lung capacity).

Closed-circuit spirometry facilitates the measurement of IC by affording the operator the capacity to scrutinise the stability of FRC during tidal breathing before asking the patient to inspire fully. Volume-displacement spirometers must contain a volume of air at the start of the manoeuvre that is greater than the patient's IC so that a full inspiratory breath can be measured.

Flow spirometers, provided they have the software to integrate inspiratory as well as expiratory flow, are usually more suitable as they do not require the patient to breathe in from an air reservoir.

THE FLOW-VOLUME CURVE OR LOOP

Measures of maximum flow can be made either absolutely (e.g. peak expiratory flow) or expressed as a function of volume, the latter by generating a flow-volume curve (expiration only) or flow-volume loop (expiration followed by inspiration—Figure 2.3). The shape of this curve is reproducible for any individual but varies considerably between different lung diseases. A poorly performed manoeuvre is usually characterised by alterations in the shape of the curve and by poor repeatability. The measurements derived from the flow-volume curve include those listed above for the spirogram and the following:

- **$FEF_{50\%}$** and **$FEF_{75\%}$** (forced expiratory flow at 50% or 75% FVC) are the maximal expiratory flow measured at the point where 50% of the FVC has been expired ($FEF_{50\%}$) and after 75% has been expired ($FEF_{75\%}$). Both indices have a wide range of normality but are usually repeatable in a given subject, provided the FVC does not vary between blows.

- **PEF** (peak expiratory flow) is the maximal expiratory flow achieved. This occurs very early in the forced expiratory manoeuvre. The PEF is an index of airflow limitation mainly due to obstruction in the large airways. The measurement of PEF is effort-dependent; therefore, the subject must perform with maximal effort otherwise it will be underestimated and poorly repeatable.

- **PIF** (peak inspiratory flow) is the maximal inspiratory flow achieved. Unlike the PEF, the PIF occurs at about midway through inspiration (i.e. about 50% FVC). The whole of the inspiratory limb of the flow-volume loop is effort-dependent; therefore, PIF varies with effort. When correctly performed, the PIF can provide useful information about fixed upper airflow obstruction.

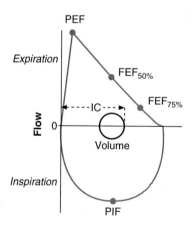

Figure 2.3 Normal maximal flow-volume loop showing the peak expiratory and inspiratory flows (PEF and PIF) and maximum flows after 50% and 75% of the FVC had been expired (FEF$_{50\%}$ and FEF$_{75\%}$). Note that in health the shape of the flow-volume curve approximates a straight-sided triangle (expiration) on top of a deep semicircle (inspiration). Healthy young subjects often have a hump on the descending portion of the expiratory curve, suggesting well-maintained airway calibre. Respiratory disease can dramatically alter the shape of the flow-volume loop.

All indices of ventilatory function (volumes and flows) should be reported at body temperature and pressure saturated with water vapour (BTPS). If this is not done, the results will be underestimated because when the patient blows into a 'cold' spirometer, the volume recorded by the spirometer is less than that displaced by the lungs. The expired gas cools to a degree dependent on the temperature inside the spirometer—normally the ambient temperature of the room (see Appendix B).

SUMMARY

Spirometry is usually recorded as either a spirogram or a flow-volume curve (or loop). The most commonly measured indices are FEV_1, FVC, FEV_1/FVC ratio, PEF and $FEF_{25-75\%}$. In addition, indices based on the 6-second forced expiration (FVC_6) and the IC (as a measure of dynamic hyperinflation) are gaining popularity. The shape of the flow-volume curve often provides very useful additional and complementary information (see Chapter 7). All measurements of volume and flow are reported after correction to BTPS conditions.

CHAPTER 3

MEASUREMENT DEVICES

Spirometers can be categorised as either volume-displacement or flow spirometers depending on whether they primarily measure volume or flow (Figure 3.1). Flow spirometers are the most commonly used and are available as full diagnostic instruments or monitors with limited functionality. The minimum performance standards for all spirometers are summarised in Appendix A (Table A.1).

Volume-displacement spirometers

rolling seal   water sealed   bellows

Flow spirometers

ultrasonic   hot-wires

pneumotachographs   pitot tube   turbine

Figure 3.1   Schematic diagrams showing examples of volume-displacement and flow spirometers. Flow spirometers have largely replaced volume-displacement spirometers, especially in general practice.

VOLUME-DISPLACEMENT SPIROMETERS

These are conventional spirometers that provide a direct measure of respired volume from the displacement of a bell (water-sealed), piston (rolling seal) or bellows (e.g. wedge bellows).

The results are normally presented as a graphic display of expired volume against time (a spirogram). The indices FEV_1, FVC and VC are generally manually calculated (including back-extrapolation (see Chapter 4) and correction to BTPS (see Appendix B)) from the spirogram by the operator, and for this reason volume-displacement spirometers are sometimes considered time-consuming and less convenient for routine use in a busy doctor's surgery. $FEF_{25-75\%}$ is also sometimes measured as an index of early disease affecting the peripheral airways (e.g. in asymptomatic smokers). Some volume-displacement spirometers are computer-assisted to reduce testing time as all computations, including correction to BTPS, are performed automatically. An important advantage of computerised volume-displacement spirometers that also incorporate a kymograph (rotating drum to move the recording paper) is that the operator can manually verify the accuracy of the computer-derived results from the simultaneously recorded spirogram.

Generally, volume-displacement spirometers are robust, simple to use, accurate, reliable, easy to maintain and provide a clear and permanent record of the test. They are, however, less portable than flow spirometers, more difficult to clean and disinfect and have relatively poor dynamic characteristics. Some do not have the capacity to measure inspiratory volumes or to compare tidal with maximal breathing. Although their dynamic response characteristics are adequate for faithful recording of events occurring over a second or more (e.g. FVC, FEV_1), they are not usually sufficiently fast to accurately record rapid events (e.g. PEF measurements). Volume spirometers have been and are still widely used in respiratory laboratories, but to a lessor extent in general practice clinics and epidemiological surveys of lung function, and are the instruments most familiar to clinicians. However, spirometers utilising flow sensors are now more popular and have advantages in terms of portability, infection control and, in many, the capacity to measure inspiratory volumes (e.g. IC, IVC, FIV_1) and to compare tidal breathing with the flow-volume loop.

FLOW SPIROMETERS

Over recent years, advances in electronics and low-cost microprocessor technology have led to the development of a wide range of flow spirometers. Flow spirometers utilise a sensor that measures flow as the primary signal and calculates volume by electronic (analogue) or numerical (digital) integration of the flow signal. The most commonly used flow sensors detect and measure flow from the pressure drop across a known, constant resistance (e.g. a pneumotachograph or orifice); the cooling of one or more heated wires (an anemometer); the transmission of ultrasonic sound waves; or by electronically counting the rotation of a turbine blade.

For the family practitioner, these devices have largely replaced the manual volume-displacement spirometer. This is because they are usually easily portable, automatically calculate all ventilatory indices, correct values to BTPS conditions, provide immediate feedback on the acceptability of each test attempted, select the best results, store patient results, calculate normal reference values and lower limit of normal for the patient being tested, and provide a print-out of the results including the spirogram and flow-volume curve. Some also provide an interpretation of the results, but the appropriateness of these comments depends on the use of correct predicted normal values and rules employed by the software to classify ventilatory defects and grade their severity.

These features, together with their lower price, ease of use and maintenance (e.g. cleaning and disinfection) have made flow-based spirometers very popular. Their capacity to measure inspiratory volumes is another major advantage.

Some flow spirometers have single patient use disposable sensors that also serve as the mouthpiece, effectively eliminating the need for cleaning and disinfection. However, the accuracy of each new sensor needs to be established. Accuracy and reproducibility depend on the stability and calibration of the electronic circuitry and appropriate correction of flow and volume to BTPS conditions (see Appendix B). For example, a small error when detecting zero flow (i.e. drift) may cause some devices to produce large errors in the measurement of FVC, as the error may be continually added during the time needed to complete the blow.

With heavy use, the sensor may also change its calibration due to the condensation of water vapour, deposition of mucus or changes in the mechanical operation of the sensor. Even the presence of the finest hair can interfere with the free rotation of a turbine or the calibration of a hot-wire anemometer. Knowledge and application of regular calibration procedures are required to detect such errors and are an essential part of the care of these machines, as they are of any other spirometer.

Further, not all flow spirometers provide flexibility in the choice of normal reference values relevant to your population or allow the operator to manually enter personally selected, predicted equations.

At present, some spirometers also limit the user's capacity to fully configure the format of the printed report, including the choice of lung function indices, and may lack customisation to include the name and address of your business.

MONITORING DEVICES AND PEAK FLOW METERS

Monitoring devices are spirometers that are suitable for frequent, repeated use for serially assessing and quantifying change in ventilatory function. Note that monitoring devices have to meet the same equipment requirements (e.g. accuracy) as diagnostic spirometers (Miller et al. 2005b) (see Appendix A). They are usually less expensive and measure a limited range of indices.

Mechanical devices for personal use by patients, such as the peak flow meter, have been available for several decades for serial monitoring of lung function and have proven useful in the management of asthma. Typically, they use the principle of airflow through a tube causing the displacement of a spring-loaded disc that in turn displaces a marker along a scale calibrated in litres per minute. Most peak flow meters are robust and provide reproducible results essential for serial monitoring. However, they often have limited accuracy and, because they provide only a single effort-dependent index of ventilatory function and do not provide a graphical display to check patient effort, they have limited application in the initial assessment of respiratory diseases.

The PEF is reduced in diseases causing airways obstruction and to a lesser extent in neuromuscular diseases in which there is reduced expiratory muscle strength. Peak flow monitoring is particularly useful for following trends in lung function, quantifying response to treatment and identifying trigger factors in asthma. This is because these devices have high precision and can detect changes in PEF.

Peak flow meters can vary considerably in accuracy between brands; this is sometimes due to the complex physical characteristics of the spring component resulting in non-linear performance. The accuracy of some peak flow meters has been enhanced through the use of a non-linear measurement scale; that is, they are calibrated to compensate for non-linearity in their physical performance.

Also available are peak flow meters that produce a whistle when the patient's PEF achieves a preset level (as set by the patient's physician). These devices are useful for children ('if you can make it whistle, then your lungs are okay'), for the vision-impaired and for quick assessment at night in the dark.

Recently, small, reliable, inexpensive yet accurate, battery-powered electronic devices for measuring ventilatory function (including FEV_1) have been developed. Some can store the test data with date and time, which can be downloaded onto a computer for review and statistical analysis. As mentioned, monitoring devices have to meet the same equipment standards as full-performance spirometers.

These devices are becoming more popular as their price decreases with increasing demand and may eventually replace the traditional peak flow meter.

CALIBRATION AND QUALITY CONTROL

Accurate and reliable spirometry requires an ongoing program of preventative maintenance that includes regular cleaning and calibration (or validation) checks to ensure that the machine is operating correctly and consistently providing clinically useful results. Most electronic spirometers incorporate a specific calibration subroutine as part of the software, whereas volume-displacement spirometers often require the calibration to be done manually. All diagnostic spirometers must be capable of being calibrated or having their calibration checked, and this should be done regularly. Be wary of claims by some manufacturers that their spirometer does not require calibration. Some models, however, have been shown to maintain their accuracy over extended periods of heavy clinical use.

3 litre calibration syringe

From a practical point of view, the accuracy of a spirometer is checked using a certified 3 litre calibration syringe and the procedure is normally carried out via a calibration subroutine. When the 3 litres is passed into the spirometer it should record a volume to within ±3.5% (Miller et al. 2005b). That is, the spirometer is accurate if the recorded volume is between 2.895 and 3.105 litres ATPS.

Flow spirometers should also be checked weekly for *linearity* over the physiological range of flows (ideally 0–14 L/s). A good test of linearity (and accuracy) is to deliver the 3 litres several times at different rates to cover a wide range of flows. If the spirometer is linear, the volume recorded by the spirometer will remain between 2.895 and 3.105 litres over the flow range (see Figure 3.2).

However, if the volume recorded falls outside these limits then the spirometer is inaccurate and may be non-linear. Records of

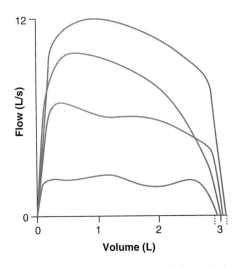

Figure 3.2 Checking the accuracy and linearity of the flow spirometer requires a 3 litre syringe to be emptied at several speeds. In this example, the spirometer is accurate over a wide flow range because the volume measured by the spirometer was always between the ATS/ERS accuracy limits of 2.895 and 3.105 litres (indicated by the dotted lines).

calibration checks, quality control and service history should be recorded in a logbook and kept with the equipment. It is important to remember that, as with any mechanical device, a calibration syringe should be checked for correct performance and accuracy periodically. Leaks can be checked easily but the accuracy of the syringe needs to be checked by the supplier or manufacturer.

Volume-displacement spirometers should be checked for volume linearity every 3 months by consecutive injections of 1-litre increments from a calibration syringe.

Leaks and timing accuracy

Volume-displacement spirometers should be checked daily for *leaks* by filling the spirometer and applying a weight to the spirometer bell (or by applying a constant pressure ≥ 3 cmH₂0 or 0.3 kPa) with breathing hoses attached and plugged, and observing any volume change. In practice, a volume change of less than 0.03 litres over a 60-second period is acceptable. If a kymograph is fitted, the *paper speed* should also be checked with a stopwatch every 3 months or immediately when an error is suspected. An error in accuracy of within 2% is acceptable.

Frequency

The frequency of performing checks will vary with the clinical setting (e.g. how often it is used) and the type of spirometer, and the need to adjust the calibration will depend on whether its accuracy is within acceptable limits. Table 3.1 provides the frequency of performing these checks as recommended by the ATS/ERS. Some spirometers are more stable than others. For example, in the absence of a leak, volume-displacement spirometers such as the rolling seal usually maintain their accuracy for extended periods and the frequency of calibration may be weekly with daily checks for leaks. However, flow spirometers generally require daily or twice-daily calibration checks. There are possible exceptions, for example, a popular ultrasonic spirometer has been shown to maintain accuracy over extended periods of heavy clinical use (Walters et al. 2006; Skloot, Edwards & Enright 2010). All spirometers must be recalibrated (or their calibration verified) after cleaning or disinfection, or if an unusual or unexpected result indicates a problem.

TABLE 3.1	Frequency of quality control
Test	**Frequency**
Volume	Daily
Leak	Daily
Volume linearity	Every 3 months
Flow linearity	Weekly
Time	Every 3 months

Source: Miller et al. (2005b).

Biological controls

In order to detect changes in overall spirometer performance, the ventilatory function of one or more subjects with stable respiratory function should be measured and recorded regularly as part of an ongoing quality control program. In the surgery, testing yourself (if you have stable lung function) on your spirometer every week is a practical way of monitoring quality control. Generally, a variation of more than 5% in FEV_1 or FVC should alert you to a problem and the need to have your instrument properly checked and serviced. A practical approach is to measure the spirometry of the subject 10 times over a period of two to three weeks. From the results, calculate the mean and standard deviation for both FEV_1 and FVC. From these calculate the 95% confidence interval (mean ±1.96 standard deviation). Any value for FEV_1 or FVC that subsequently falls outside these limits should alert you to the possibility that the spirometer has become inaccurate. The easiest way to handle serial data of this type is to plot it as a Levy–Jennings diagram, as shown in Figure 3.3. Remember that testing a normal subject does not negate the need to calibrate (or to check the calibration of) the instrument regularly using a certified 3 litre syringe.

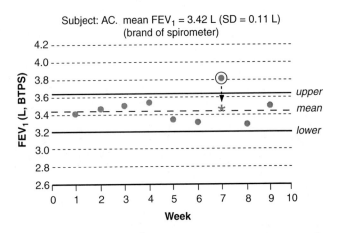

Figure 3.3 Plotting serial results from a normal control subject allows 'out of control' values to be identified easily. The upper and lower limits were calculated from the mean ±1.96 × standard deviation (see text). Here the FEV_1 at week 7 is outside the expected range and alerts you to a potential problem. In this example, recalibration of the spirometer with a 3 litre syringe brings the FEV_1 back into the acceptable range (asterisk).

BTPS correction

It should be noted that if the accuracy of the spirometer is checked with a 3 litre syringe while the spirometer is in 'patient' rather than 'calibration' mode (if available), the volume recorded will usually be higher than the expected accuracy range of 2.895 to 3.105 litres.

This is because in the patient-testing mode the spirometer will apply the BTPS correction factor (and possibly other factors, for example, correction for gas viscosity). For a computerised volume-displacement spirometer, the recorded volume will be about 3.3 litres if the room temperature is 20°C.

When a volume-displacement spirometer is moved into a cooler or hotter environment, it is important to allow time for it to reach the new temperature and to measure it, otherwise the BTPS correction factor (see Appendix B) will be incorrect. Similarly, the calibration syringe needs to be at the same temperature as the spirometer and for this reason it is usually stored with the spirometer.

Mechanical peak flow meters can generally be expected to wear out after about 12 to 24 months of heavy use, although there is little published data to support this. However, a volume-displacement spirometer will usually last many years if properly maintained and serviced.

FACTORS TO CONSIDER WHEN CHOOSING A SPIROMETER

Factors governing the choice of spirometer for use in a doctor's surgery include (Burton, Johns & Swanney 2005):

- ease of use
- provision of easy-to-read real-time graphic display of the manoeuvre
- provision of immediate quality feedback concerning the acceptability of blows, including repeatability
- provision to interface with clinical software packages
- provision of customisable final spirometry report
- provision to print the final report
- price and running costs
- reliability and ease of maintenance
- training, servicing and repair of the spirometer provided by the supplier
- ability to trial the spirometer in your setting before you purchase
- provision of a disposable sensor or a breathing circuit that can be easily cleaned and disinfected
- provision of appropriate normal reference values with lower limits of normal
- robustness
- provision of a comprehensive manual describing its operation, maintenance and calibration

- calibration requirements
- conforms to accepted spirometry performance standards (Appendix A)
- complies with electrical safety standards.

A summary of the specifications and features of spirometers on the market in Australia and New Zealand is provided in the *Spirometers Users' and Buyers' Guide* (Burton, Johns & Swanney 2011) available at www.nationalasthma.org.au.

Faced with the wide variety of spirometers available today, general practitioners have to choose an instrument suitable for use in their own surgery. If possible, trial the spirometer before buying to ensure it meets *your* specific needs.

SUMMARY

All spirometers are regarded as diagnostic instruments and should meet or exceed relevant ATS/ERS equipment standards. Spirometers must be capable of being calibrated, or at least having their calibration checked, to ensure their ongoing accuracy. A certified 3 litre syringe is recommended for calibrating spirometers, and this should be done regularly and the results recorded. To assess overall spirometer performance it is recommended that biological controls be included in the spirometer's quality assurance program with the results recorded in a table and Levy–Jennings plot. When purchasing a spirometer it is important that it meets or exceeds minimum performance criteria.

CHAPTER 4

HOW TO DO SPIROMETRY AND THE COMMON PROBLEMS

HOW TO DO SPIROMETRY

To ensure an acceptable result, the FVC manoeuvre must be performed with maximum effort immediately following a maximum inspiration; it should have a rapid start and the spirogram or flow-volume curve should be a smooth continuous curve throughout the manoeuvre. The test can be tiring for the elderly or breathless patient, so sufficient time for recovery should be allowed between repeat tests. It is important that the operator is properly trained before attempting to measure spirometry.

There are two breathing circuits commonly used when performing spirometry: closed- and open-circuit methods (Figure 4.1). The *open-circuit* method is used when the subject inspires fully before going onto the mouthpiece to perform the forced manoeuvre. The *closed-circuit* method requires the subject to first breathe tidally on the mouthpiece and then to inspire fully from the spirometer before performing the forced manoeuvre. The latter method has the advantage that the subject's inspired volume can be measured and is displayed, which can help to verify that the subject has inspired fully prior to performing the forced manoeuvre, and also has the advantage of being able to compare tidal with maximal breathing.

To achieve good results, carefully explain to the patient the procedure (be clear and precise) and what is being measured. Also ensure that he or she is sitting upright with feet firmly on the floor (the safest and most comfortable position; although standing and sitting give a similar result in adults, in children the VC is usually

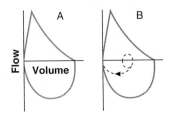

Figure 4.1 Open and closed circuit. The flow-volume loop performed by the open-circuit (A) and closed-circuit (B) methods (see text). When correctly performed the results for both methods are the same. However, the closed-circuit method has the advantage that tidal breathing can be displayed and it is easier to verify that the subject had fully inspired before commencing the forced expiratory manoeuvre. Only the closed-circuit method allows IC to be measured.

---

greater in the standing position). A nose clip must be worn when measuring IC and inspiratory VC and when performing a slow VC manoeuvre and is recommended when performing a forced (FVC) manoeuvre. A nose clip is not needed when measuring PEF. Do not use a chair with wheels. Remember that verbal encouragement/ coaching throughout the test is essential.

Open-circuit spirometry

Demonstrate the manoeuvre to the patient. Apply a nose clip to the patient's nose (this is recommended, but not essential) and urge the patient to:

- breathe in fully (the subject should inspire rapidly until absolutely full)
- seal his or her lips around the mouthpiece and *immediately blast* the air out as fast and as far as possible until the lungs are *completely* empty (the patient should remain upright)
- breathe in again as forcibly and fully as possible (not all spirometers will measure inspiration).

Obtain at least three acceptable tests and *then* apply the repeatability criteria (Table 4.1, p. 27).

The measurement of IC using open-circuit spirometry involves switching the patient into this circuit at the end of quiet expiration (i.e. FRC) and measuring the maximum volume that can be inspired (i.e. to TLC).

Closed-circuit spirometry

Demonstrate the manoeuvre to the patient. Apply a nose clip to the patient's nose (this is recommended, but not essential) and urge the patient to:

- seal his or her lips around the mouthpiece
- breath tidally for 2 to 4 breaths—usually until a stable FRC is recorded
- breathe in fully (the subject should inspire rapidly until absolutely full) and *immediately blast* the air out as fast and as far as possible until the lungs are *completely* empty (the patient should remain upright)
- breathe in again as forcibly and fully as possible (not all spirometers will measure inspiration).

Obtain at least three acceptable tests and *then* apply the repeatability criteria (Table 4.1, p. 27).

Closed-circuit spirometry facilitates the measurement of IC by affording the operator the capacity to scrutinise the stability of FRC during tidal breathing before asking the patient to inspire fully. Volume-displacement spirometers must contain a volume of air at the start of the manoeuvre that is greater than the patient's IC so that a full inspiratory breath can be measured.

Flow spirometers, provided they have the software to integrate inspiratory as well as expiratory flow, are usually more suitable as they do not require the patient to breathe in from an air reservoir.

Essentials of both open- and closed-circuit spirometry

For both methods, the *essentials* are:

- maximal inspiration
- a good seal between the lips and mouthpiece
- very vigorous effort right from the start of the manoeuvre, continuing until *absolutely* no more air can be exhaled
- rapid start
- the patient avoiding coughing, tongue occlusion, glottis closure, premature termination of the blow, etc. (see below)
- the patient not leaning forward during the test.

See also Table 4.1 (on p. 27).

The operator should be confident that the patient has followed the instructions. Note that failure to initially fill the lungs is a very common cause of poor quality spirometry.

Because the initial part of the expiration and all of the inspiration is effort-dependent, it is essential to achieve maximum patient effort in the performance of spirometry. Demonstrating to the patient the vigour and effort required is perhaps the best way to achieve this.

If only PEF is being measured, the patient need only exhale for a couple of seconds.

Remember that, particularly in patients with airflow obstruction, it may take the patient many seconds to fully exhale. It is also important to recognise those patients whose efforts are submaximal. There is no substitute for careful explanation and demonstration—demonstrating the manoeuvre to the patient will overcome 90% of problems encountered and can be critical in achieving satisfactory results. Observation and encouragement of the patient's performance are also crucial. Be sure to examine the spirogram (or flow-volume curve) for acceptability and repeatability (see below) and, if your spirometer doesn't do this for you, to correct the measurements to BTPS conditions (see Appendix B).

MEASUREMENTS IN YOUNG CHILDREN

The measurement of spirometry in young children is a particular challenge and usually limited to those 4–5 years of age and older. It is important to present the child with a non-threatening environment, to minimise interruptions, to capture the child's imagination and to make spirometry fun. The instructions must be kept short and simple. Use body language and voice intonations to reinforce your instructions. Use very simple and understandable words and phrases such as 'blow like the big wolf' or 'blow the biggest mountain' and point to the flow-volume loop on the screen. Avoid words like 'inhale' and 'maximum' as a child may never have experienced these. As with adults, it usually helps to demonstrate the test. Children who are unable to perform satisfactory spirometry on their first visit often perform the test correctly at the next visit.

ACCEPTABILITY AND REPEATABILITY CRITERIA

At least three technically acceptable manoeuvres should be obtained which meet the ATS/ERS acceptability and repeatability criteria given in Table 4.1. It is important that the acceptability criteria be applied and unacceptable tests discarded *before* assessing repeatability, as the latter is used to determine whether additional tests from the three acceptable ones already obtained are required. These criteria (together with a properly maintained and calibrated spirometer) help to ensure the quality of your results, which is essential when comparing results with predicted values and quantifying change over time. Tests that do not fully meet the acceptability criteria may still be clinically useful. For example, FEV_1 may still be valid if cough or premature termination of the blow occurs after the first second. The report should state when the results are obtained from manoeuvres that do not meet acceptability and repeatability criteria.

TABLE 4.1	Acceptability and repeatability criteria

Each individual test is acceptable if it meets the following criteria:

Start of test criteria (apply to each test)

- There was no evidence of hesitation.

- The test was performed with a rapid start (i.e. the extrapolated volume is less than 5% or 0.15 L, whichever is greater).

- The PEF has a sharp rise (flow-volume).

End of test criteria (apply to each test)

- Expiration continued until there was no change in volume (< 0.025 L) for ≥ 1 second, and the patient had blown for ≥ 3 seconds (children aged < 10 years) or for ≥ 6 seconds (subjects aged ≥ 10 years).

- (However, the patient or person conducting the test can terminate the blow if the patient cannot or should not continue.)

Other criteria (apply to each test)

- The patient followed instructions.

- A continuous maximal expiratory manoeuvre throughout the test (i.e. no stops and starts) was achieved and was initiated from full inspiration.

- There were no leaks.

- No cough (note FEV_1 may be valid if cough occurs after the first second).

- No glottis closure (Valsalva).

- No obstruction of the mouthpiece (e.g. by the tongue or teeth).

- No premature termination (note FEV_1 may be valid if this occurs after the first second).

- No evidence that the patient took an additional breath during the expiratory manoeuvre.

4

Table 4.1 continued

Repeatability criteria
• Obtain three acceptable tests (i.e. each test should meet the above acceptability criteria).
• The two largest values for FEV_1 should agree to within 0.15 litre.
• The two largest values for FVC should agree to within 0.15 litre.
• Repeat the test if these repeatability criteria are not met.
Results to report
• FEV_1—report the largest value.
• FVC—report the largest value.
• PEF—report the largest value.
• FEV_6—report the largest value.
• $FEF_{25-75\%}$—report the value obtained from the test with highest sum of FEV_1 + FVC.

Source: Miller et al. (2005b).

BACK-EXTRAPOLATION

Back-extrapolation is a procedure applied to the volume versus time curve to determine the appropriate time zero from which all timed volumes (e.g. FEV_1) are calculated . The derived time zero is the point on the time axis where exhalation would have started assuming 'instantaneous' flow acceleration (i.e. the patient's maximal flow is projected back to the volume axis). The procedure minimises errors in the measurement of FEV_1 if the expiratory manoeuvre was not performed rapidly from the very start.

Back-extrapolation is quite simple. To calculate time zero, draw a line through the steepest portion of the volume-time curve and extend it back to the time axis. This point is taken as time zero (Figure 4.2). From this construction the 'extrapolated volume' can be calculated as shown in Figure 4.2. For an acceptably rapid start to the blow, the ATS/ERS requires that the extrapolated volume should be less than 5% FVC or 0.15 litres, whichever is greater. An extrapolated volume higher than this indicates that the blow was not initiated sufficiently rapidly and should be repeated.

The back-extrapolation procedure is performed by hand with manual spirometers; however, in practice this is often only done when the spirogram shows an obvious slow start (i.e. measurable

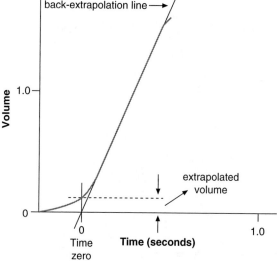

Figure 4.2 The back-extrapolation procedure to determine time zero and the extrapolated volume.

extrapolated volume). Computerised spirometers that meet ATS/ERS equipment standards (Miller et al. 2005b) will perform this procedure automatically, and many will provide immediate feedback if the extrapolated volume exceeds acceptable limits (i.e. 5% FVC or 0.15 litres, whichever is greater).

PATIENT-RELATED PROBLEMS

It is useful to learn how to recognise inadequacies in the performance of spirometry and the recordings as these can greatly affect the accuracy, repeatability and hence interpretation of the results. Figures 4.3 and 4.4 show some problematic examples compared with well-performed manoeuvres, illustrated for both the expiratory spirogram and the flow-volume loop respectively.

As stated, optimum patient performance is crucial to obtaining valid spirometry. The patient must understand fully that the manoeuvre *must* be performed with maximal effort. If the test is performed correctly, the results from repeat blows will usually be reproducible (i.e. FEV_1 and FVC to within 0.15 litres).

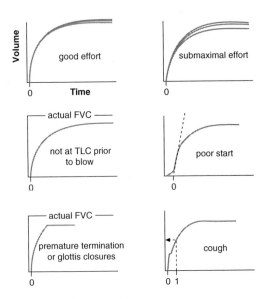

Figure 4.3 Common problems in the performance of spirometry are shown on these expiratory spirograms.

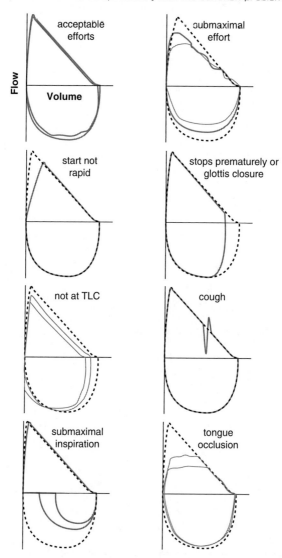

Figure 4.4 Common problems in the performance of spirometry are shown in these flow-volume loops. The dotted flow-volume loop represents the acceptable maximal effort.

The most common patient-related problems when performing the FVC manoeuvre are:

- submaximal effort
- leaks between the lips and mouthpiece
- incomplete inspiration or expiration (prior to or during the forced manoeuvre)
- hesitation at the start of the expiration
- cough (particularly within the first second of expiration)
- glottis closure causing an abrupt reduction in flow or straight sections (rather than a smooth curve) in the spirogram
- obstruction of the mouthpiece by the tongue or teeth (false or otherwise)
- vocalisation during the forced manoeuvre
- poor posture.

These problems can largely be avoided by giving the patient clear instructions with *vigorous* verbal reinforcement throughout the test. Demonstration of the procedure will also help prevent many of these problems, remembering that all effort-dependent measurements will be variable in patients who are uncooperative or deliberately trying to produce low values.

Failure to empty the lungs completely (premature termination) is very common, resulting in an underestimation of both FVC and exaggerated evidence of airflow obstruction (overestimated FEV_1/FVC ratio). To avoid this, active encouragement right to the end of the blow is essential. The FVC can be greatly overestimated (and FEV_1/FVC underestimated) if the patient manages to take an extra breath through the nose during the expiratory manoeuvre (see Figure 4.5).

Glottis closure should be suspected if flow ceases or falls abruptly during the test rather than being a continuous smooth curve. Recordings in which cough, particularly if this occurs within the first second (it may affect the FEV_1), or hesitation at the start has occurred should be rejected. Vocalisation during the test will reduce flows and must be discouraged; performing the manoeuvre with the neck extended often helps.

Chest pain, abdominal problems, fear of incontinence or even just lack of confidence or embarrassment may reduce patient effort. Nose clips are recommended but are not essential when performing forced manoeuvres. Discourage the patient from leaning forward during testing; it may be helpful to tape a target to the opposite wall.

Modifying the cardboard mouthpiece, as shown below in Figure 4.6, can generally prevent obstruction of the mouthpiece by the tongue. The end of the mouthpiece is cut or shaped at an angle of about

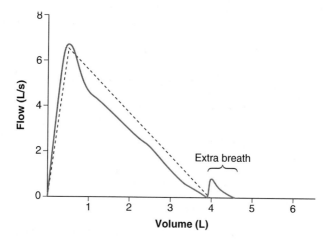

Figure 4.5 Example of a patient taking an extra breath through the nose towards the end of the expiration. The FVC is overestimated and FEV_1/FVC underestimated. The dotted line is the predicted curve.

Figure 4.6 Most mouthpieces can be modified as shown to eliminate occlusion of the mouthpiece by the tongue. Note that the sloped face of the mouthpiece must be positioned as shown.

60° to its length and used with the *sloped side upward*, preventing obstruction by the tongue. Alternatively, the problem can be reduced significantly by instructing the subject to place the mouthpiece well into the mouth and to bite it lightly.

INSTRUMENT-RELATED PROBLEMS

These depend largely on the type of spirometer used but generally the most common problems are:

- leaks in the spirometer, breathing hose and hose connections, and timing inaccuracies (in volume-displacement spirometers)
- rips and tears in the flowhead connector tube and clogged sensor (in flow spirometers)
- calibration, accuracy, signal drift and linearity (in flow spirometers).

Standards recommend checking the calibration at least daily with a calibrated syringe; a simple self-test of the spirometer is an additional, useful daily check that the instrument is functioning correctly. Other faults may require repair by the manufacturer or distributor.

When using the volume-displacement spirometer that has a limited time axis (e.g. the Vitalograph spirometer), it is very important to continue to record expired volume until the patient's lungs are empty and not to discontinue once the chart carrier stops moving, otherwise you will underestimate FVC and overestimate the FEV_1/FVC ratio. When using a volume-displacement spirometer that utilises a rotating drum (kymograph) to move the recording paper, it is important to allow the paper to reach the correct speed before the patient begins to blow. Therefore, switch on the kymograph a second or two before the patient blows.

PERFORMING SPIROMETRY IN THE BUSY CLINICAL PRACTICE

There is no doubt that spirometry is time-consuming, requiring about 20 minutes to perform, document and interpret pre- and post-bronchodilator measurements. This, together with the cost of purchasing and maintaining a spirometer, are arguments often put by general practitioners for not including spirometry as part of their general practice consultations.

There are a number of ways to make testing more cost-effective (Fardy 2001):

- Perform pre-bronchodilator spirometry as soon as you have determined that your patient's problems may be related to asthma or COPD. Administer a bronchodilator and then complete the history-taking and clinical examination. By the time you have done this, sufficient time (10 minutes or more) will have passed for the post-bronchodilator blows to be done. With the results of spirometry now available, you will be better equipped to discuss the diagnosis, outlook and management plan with your patient. This strategy adds only about 10 minutes to your consultation but adds a lot of information that will be of immediate value and provide baseline measurements for future comparison (e.g. effect-iveness of treatment).
- Your practice nurse can measure the patient's spirometry for you, provided he or she has completed a comprehensive training course in spirometry.

SUMMARY

4

Acceptable spirometry requires close cooperation between the patient and the operator in the performance of maximal breathing manoeuvres. Clear and concise instructions with constant encour-agement from the operator are essential to obtain accurate and reproducible results. This is especially challenging in young children. At least three technically acceptable tests should be obtained and the FEV_1 and FVC in two of the three tests should vary by less than 0.15 litres. The highest FEV_1 and FVC (even if from separate blows) are reported. The quoted $FEF_{25-75\%}$ should be calculated from the single blow with the highest sum of FEV_1 plus FVC. A range of patient- and instrument-related problems can affect the results but most of these can be easily identified and avoided.

CHAPTER 5

INFECTION CONTROL

CROSS-INFECTION AND LUNG FUNCTION TESTING

Although there is little evidence of direct transmission of disease via lung function equipment, there is evidence that pathogenic organisms can contaminate lung function equipment thus posing a risk of cross-infection between patients (Unstead et al. 2006; Miller et al. 2005a). During spirometry patients can generate flows up to 14 L/s (840 L/min), which can easily mobilise saliva and create dense macro- and micro-aerosols by entrainment of the fluid lining the mucous membranes. These can then be deposited in the equipment and connecting tubing. Unless such deposition is prevented or the equipment is rigorously cleaned and decontaminated between patients, the chance of cross-infection exists. This is particularly important today where our patients range from healthy to the more immunosuppressed (due to illness or treatment) where the likelihood of cross-infection may be increased.

Although the transmission of respiratory pathogens (e.g. *Mycobacterium avium*, *M. tuberculosis* and the *Aspergillus* species) via spirometers has not been fully established, the potential risks are difficult to disprove. However, it has been established that organisms such as *Pseudomonas*, *Burkholderia cepacia*, *Haemophilus influenzae* and acid-fast bacillae can be recovered from spirometers.

A comprehensive review of the potential sources and risks of cross-infection during lung function testing and the methods available for disinfection and sterilisation and practical recommendations have been published (see Kendrick, Johns & Leeming 2003).

REDUCING THE RISK OF CROSS-INFECTION

Hand washing after each patient is the most effective measure to prevent nasocomial infections. Hot soapy water using an antiseptic soap is recommended.

In patients with a known infectious disease, many laboratories prefer to measure ventilatory function using a pneumotachograph or other electronic flow-sensors, as these can usually be more easily and effectively cleaned and sterilised than conventional bellows or water-sealed spirometers, which have nooks and crannies in which organisms may flourish. Since it is usually impractical to decontaminate the interior surfaces of a spirometer between patients effectively, most lung function laboratories clean and disinfect their equipment periodically (weekly or monthly). The efficacy of decontamination protocols at reducing the risk of cross-infection has not been documented and the risk certainly remains if decontamination of the equipment is not carried out after each patient. Spirometers will usually require recalibration (or that the calibration be checked) after cleaning and decontamination.

If you are disassembling the spirometer for cleaning, it is essential to:

- thoroughly clean and decontaminate the components
- thoroughly dry the components before reassembling
- check the spirometer for correct operation
- check and, if necessary, adjust the calibration.

Mouthpieces must be disposed of or cleaned and disinfected between patients because the greatest danger of cross-infection is via direct contact with bodily fluids.

An alternative approach that is now widespread is the use of a disposable (single patient use) barrier filter. This is attached to the mouthpiece of the spirometer and the patient performs the breathing manoeuvre through it to minimise the risk of equipment contamination. These filters have a low resistance to flow and have been shown not to significantly affect the clinical measurements of ventilatory function, except perhaps PEF (Johns et al. 1995). The effectiveness of some of these filters at removing bacteria and viruses has been questioned, particularly when used with patients who can generate high flows (more than 700 L/min). The best filter medium available has been shown to offer a 99.7% filtration efficiency, which implies more than 99.99% cross-contamination reduction efficiency. This is probably a similar degree of protection to that offered by wet cleaning and decontaminating equipment between patients. Recent studies have shown that barrier filters are effective at preventing the contamination and hence reducing the risk of cross-infection during lung function testing (Jacques et al. 1998; Unstead et al. 2006; Bracci et al. 2011). Filters also have the advantage of protecting delicate sensors and the internal surfaces of the spirometer from damage, and they reduce the corroding effects of cleaning agents and disinfectants. The extent to which the use of filters can effectively obviate the need for cleaning and disinfection is unclear. The cost of filters may be less than the cleaning and disinfection costs, particularly in the setting of a lung function laboratory (Side et al. 1999).

Other laboratories use disposable mouthpieces containing a one-way valve to prevent inspiration from equipment; such disposable mouthpieces cannot be used with spirometers requiring an initial period of tidal breathing. However, they can be used only when performing solely expiratory spirometry and it is doubtful that they would be effective at reducing the risk of cross-infection. When using one-way mouthpieces, it is important to ensure that the patient has *fully* inspired *before* placing the mouthpiece in the mouth, as further inspiration will be prevented.

Studies documenting the risk of developing clinically relevant infection from spirometry equipment and the extent to which cleaning, disinfection or the use of filters are protective are urgently needed to provide an evidence base for clinical practice.

SUMMARY

Although there is little direct evidence of disease transmission via lung function equipment, precautions should be taken to minimise any risk. Mouthpieces must either be cleaned and disinfected between patients, or discarded. The interior and exterior surfaces of the spirometer should be decontaminated regularly. An alternative approach, which is becoming common practice in some countries, is the use of disposable, low-resistance barrier filters, which have the additional function of protecting the equipment. Also, disposable mouthpieces incorporating a one-way valve are used when only expiratory manoeuvres are performed to prevent the patient inspiring from the spirometer.

CHAPTER 6

PREDICTED NORMAL VALUES

NORMAL VALUES

To interpret ventilatory function tests in any individual, their results need to be compared with reference values obtained from a well-defined population of normal subjects matched for gender, age, height and ethnic origin, using:

- similar test protocols, and
- carefully calibrated and validated instruments.

Normal predicted values for ventilatory function generally vary as follows:

- **Gender**: For a given height and age, males have a larger FEV_1, FVC, $FEF_{25-75\%}$ and PEF but a slightly lower FEV_1/FVC ratio.
- **Age**: FEV_1, FVC, $FEF_{25-75\%}$ and PEF increase with age until about 18 years in females and 20 years in males. After this, all indices gradually fall, although the precise rate of decline is probably masked due to the complex interrelationship between age and height. The fall in the FEV_1/FVC ratio with age in adults is due to the greater decline in FEV_1 than in FVC. A large change in predicted values can occur at the transition from adolescent to adult when predicted data is obtained from separate studies.
- **Height**: All indices other than the FEV_1/FVC ratio increase with standing height. Arm span (fingertip to fingertip) may be used if the subject is unable to stand or has spinal deformity.
- **Ethnic origin**: For a given age and height, Caucasians have the largest FEV_1 and FVC and of the various ethnic groups Polynesians

are among the lowest. The values for black Africans are 10–15% lower than for Caucasians of similar age, gender and height because for a given standing height their thorax is shorter. Australian Aborigines have predicted values about 15% lower than Caucasians. Chinese have been found to have an FVC about 20% lower and Indians about 10% lower than matched Caucasians. There is little difference in PEF between ethnic groups. The FEV_1/FVC ratio is similar between ethnic groups. Many lung function laboratories use Caucasian predicted values and apply a factor (e.g. X 0.88) to approximately correct for ethnic differences.

Body weight is not a strong predictor of lung size except in subjects who are significantly under- or overweight, in which case it is usually low.

There is a vast literature of normal population studies, many of which have deficiencies in sample size, ethnicity, definition of normality, inclusion of smokers and choice of equipment. The most appropriate predicted values will be influenced by the community in which you are working. In the absence of population-specific reference values, Mediterranean values are better predicted by European ones and Australian values are better predicted by American ones.

Appendix C provides tables of mean predicted values and lower limits of normal (LLN) for Caucasians of both genders for FEV_1, FVC, FEV_1/FVC, $FEF_{25-75\%}$, PEF, FVC_6, FEV_1/FVC_6 and $FEF_{25-75\%6}$. The reference data for FEV_1, FVC, FEV_1/FVC and $FEF_{25-75\%}$ are based on the work of Stanojevic et al. (2009), who collated normal reference data from several paediatric studies and integrated them with data from the Third National Health and Nutrition Examination Survey (NHANES III) (Hankinson, Odencrantz & Fedan 1999) to produce *continuous all-age prediction equations* from age 4 to 80 years based on height and age. The adult reference data for indices based on a 6-second forced expiration (FVC_6, FEV_1/FVC_6 and $FEF_{25-75\%6}$) were compiled from data published by Hankinson, Crapo and Jensen (2003). Predicted PEF values for adults and children (aged 8–80 years) were from Hankinson, Odencrantz and Fedan (1999).

Normal values for IC can be obtained by subtracting predicted FRC from predicted TLC. Suitable reference equations for predicting FRC and TLC are available from Quanjer et al. (1993).

It is not recommended to extrapolate beyond the age and height range of the normal population used to obtain the reference equations used.

Ventilatory abnormalities can be inferred if any of FEV_1, FVC, PEF and the FEV_1/FVC ratio are below the lower limit of normal. The *lower* limit of normal can be defined by the 95% confidence interval, which for normally distributed data is 1.64 standard errors below the mean predicted value for these indices (i.e. 5% of the healthy population will be classified as abnormal). An *upper* limit of normal is not usually used for FEV_1, FVC and PEF because *disease usually only decreases* their value. For the FEV_1/FVC ratio, disease can both increase and decrease it, so the normal *range* is sometimes used as mean ±1.96 standard deviations. The use of a fixed value for the lower limit (e.g. 80% of the mean predicted for FEV_1 and FVC, and 0.70 for the FEV_1/FVC ratio) is *not recommended,* as this can result in false positives in older people and false negatives in young adults. This is illustrated in Figures 6.1 and 6.2 for FEV_1 and the FEV_1/FVC ratio respectively, where the use of a fixed lower limit value (dotted line in these figures) is clearly inappropriate.

SUMMARY

The results of spirometry (e.g. FEV_1, FVC) are usually compared with predicted values based on the patient's age, height, gender and ethnic origin. Most computerised diagnostic spirometers allow the operator to select from a number of normal value studies and some allow custom equations to be entered. A set of predicted values (lookup tables) is given in Appendix C.

6

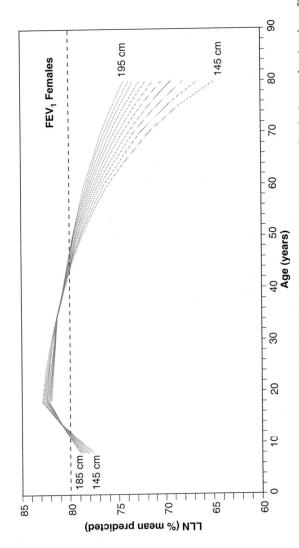

Figure 6.1 The lower limit of normal (LLN) for FEV$_1$ (females) expressed as a per cent of the mean predicted value as a function of age. This plot clearly demonstrates that the use of a fixed value for the LLN (e.g. 80% predicted—dotted line) is inappropriate, particularly for short older people. (Calculated from data published by Hankinson, Odencrantz & Fedan 1999.)

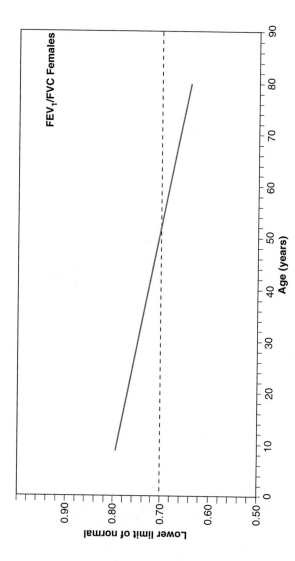

Figure 6.2 The lower limit of normal (LLN) for the FEV_1/FVC ratio (females) as a function of age (all heights). This plot clearly shows that the use of a fixed value for the LLN (e.g. 0.70—dotted line) is inappropriate. (Calculated from data published by Hankinson, Odencrantz & Fedan 1999.)

CHAPTER 7

INTERPRETATION OF SPIROMETRY

Measurements of ventilatory function may be very useful in a diagnostic sense but they are also useful in following the natural history of disease over a period of time, assessing preoperative risk and quantifying the effects of treatment. The presence of ventilatory abnormality can be inferred if one or more of FEV_1, VC, $FEF_{25-75\%}$, PEF or the FEV_1/FVC ratio is below the normal range or in the presence of an abnormal shape of the flow-volume loop.

SIGNIFICANT CHANGE IN SPIROMETRY WITH TIME

Serial measurements of ventilatory function can provide important information about disease progression and response to therapy. However, it is often difficult to decide what constitutes a significant change as this varies depending on the index (FEV_1, FVC, etc.) and the time interval between repeat measurements, and may differ in disease and healthy subjects. Table 7.1 provides recommended guidelines as to what constitutes a significant change over several time periods (Pellegrino et al. 2005).

Thus, changes greater than those given in Table 7.1 would need to occur to have confidence that the change was real. The ATS/ERS suggest that for FEV_1 short-term changes of > 12% and > 0.2 litre may be clinically important. This would be particularly true if on each occasion spirometry met the acceptability criteria and the FEV_1 was repeatable. This illustrates the importance of obtaining measurements of high quality.

TABLE 7.1	Percentage changes required to be significant	
	FVC	**FEV$_1$**
Day to day		
Normal subjects	≥ 5	≥ 5
COPD	≥ 11	≥ 13
Week to week		
Normal subjects	≥ 11	≥ 12
COPD	≥ 20	≥ 20
Year to year	≥ 15	≥ 15

Source: Pellegrino et al. (2005).

The rate of fall of FEV$_1$ over time is an important indicator of disease progression in people with COPD. In healthy, non-smoking adults the decrease is about 30 mL/year with an upper limit of about 50 mL/year. A decrease greater than this suggests an abnormally rapid rate of deterioration, presumably due to the progression of the disease. However, determining the rate of decline in a patient is not easy because it requires monitoring over years and can be greatly affected by changes in equipment performance and the quality of spirometry.

CLASSIFYING ABNORMAL VENTILATORY FUNCTION

There are three classifications for abnormal ventilatory function (see Table 7.2 and Figure 7.1):

TABLE 7.2	Classification of ventilatory abnormalities by spirometry		
	Obstructive	**Apparent restrictive**	**Mixed**
FEV$_1$	↓	↓ or N	↓
FVC	↓ or N	↓	↓
FEV$_1$/FVC	↓	↑ or N	↓

7

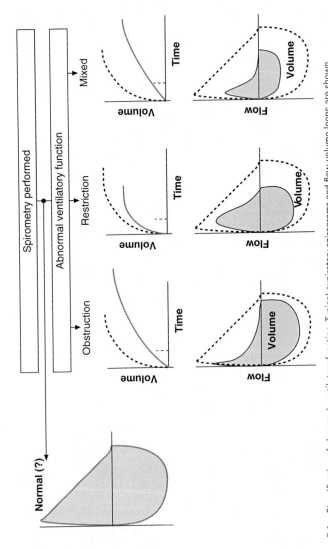

Figure 7.1 Classification of abnormal ventilatory function. Typical expiratory spirograms and flow-volume loops are shown.

1. **Obstructive ventilatory defect:** characterised by airflow limitation; for example, reduced FEV_1, FEV_1/FVC ratio or PEF. An FEV_1/FVC ratio below the lower limit of normal is often used to *detect* obstruction and the FEV_1 expressed as a per cent of the mean predicted value to *grade* its severity. (The term 'obstructive' is often used in this book as it is in common use. 'Airflow limitation' is a more accurate term as it recognises that reduced expiratory flows may be a consequence not only of airway narrowing (due to airway wall inflammation, mucus and so on) but also of dynamic airway collapse due to loss of radial traction to the airway wall as a consequence of parenchymal destruction.)

2. **Restrictive ventilatory defect:** characterised by loss of lung volume in the absence of airflow limitation, as suggested by a low VC or FVC but normal or high FEV_1/FVC ratio.

3. **Mixed obstructive and restrictive ventilatory defect:** characterised by both airflow limitation *and* loss of lung volume; that is, a low FEV_1/FVC ratio and low VC. Total lung capacity needs to be measured to confirm the restrictive component because loss of FVC and VC can occur in the presence of hyperinflation in diseases causing airflow limitation.

The interrelationships between the various measurements are important diagnostically (see Table 7.2 and Figures 7.1 and 7.2). For example:

- A reduction of FEV_1 in relation to the FVC will result in a low FEV_1/FVC ratio and is typical of *obstructive ventilatory defects* (e.g. asthma, chronic airways disease and emphysema). The lower limit of normal for the FEV_1/FVC ratio is around 0.70 but the exact lower limit is dependent on age, as shown in Figure 6.2 for females. The predicted normal values by age, gender and height are given in the tables in Appendix C. In obstructive lung disease, the FVC may be less than the slow VC because of airway closure occurring earlier during the forced manoeuvre. This may lead to an overestimation of the ratio. Thus, the FEV_1/VC ratio may be a more sensitive index for identifying airflow obstruction. It has been shown that in patients with known lung disease a reduced FEV_1/VC ratio predicts morbidity and mortality even when the FEV_1 is normal. However, in healthy people the meaning of a low ratio in the presence of a normal FEV_1 is uncertain (Pellegrino et al. 2005).

An *obstructive ventilatory defect* may also be inferred if the $FEF_{25-75\%}$ is less than the lower limit of normal, even if the FEV_1 is normal. This result suggests that the site of obstruction is the

Figure 7.2 Plot of FVC or VC (spirometric index of lung 'size'), expressed as percentage predicted, and the FEV_1/FVC ratio (index of obstruction) to illustrate the interpretation of spirometry. The vertical dotted line represents the patient's (male, aged 60 years, height 170 cm) lower limit of normal for FEV_1/FVC ratio (varies with age and gender; see Figure 6.2) and the horizontal dotted line is the lower limit of normal for FVC or VC (varies with age, gender and height). The position of the curved dotted line can vary but illustrates that with increasing airflow obstruction the FVC (or VC) is often reduced due to excessive airway narrowing and closure during the forced expiration and not due to 'small' lungs.

peripheral or small airways. It should be noted that the $FEF_{25-75\%}$ can be confidently compared with predicted normal values only if the FVC is normal. Similarly, serial measurements of $FEF_{25-75\%}$ are meaningful only if the FVC remains constant. Prolongation of the FET is also an indication of airflow obstruction.

- The FEV_1/FVC ratio remains normal or high (typically, more than 0.80) with a reduction in both FEV_1 and FVC in *restrictive ventilatory defects* (e.g. interstitial lung disease, respiratory muscle weakness and thoracic cage deformities such as kyphoscoliosis). The FEV_1/FVC ratio may also be slightly low in tall, lean and healthy subjects whose chest is long and narrow. The cause is unclear, but it may be because airway calibre is a function of chest diameter; thus the airways in these subjects may be slightly narrower than normal and limit the FEV_1.
- Alternatively, it may be a consequence of reduced growth of the airways relative to the lung parenchyma or alveolar tissue.

- A reduced FVC together with a low FEV_1/FVC ratio is a feature of a *mixed ventilatory defect* in which a combination of both obstruction and restriction appears to be present. Alternatively, this may occur in airflow obstruction as a consequence of airway closure resulting in gas trapping, rather than as a result of small lungs. It is necessary to measure the patient's total lung capacity to distinguish between these two possibilities and to quantify the restrictive component.

The shape of the expiratory flow-volume curve varies between *obstructive ventilatory defects*, where maximal flows are diminished and the expiratory curve is scooped out or convex towards the flow and volume axes, and *restrictive diseases*, where expiratory flows may be increased in relation to lung volume and the shape often convex away from the axes. Diminished flows on the expiratory curve as residual volume is approached are suggestive of obstruction in the small peripheral airways. Examination of the shape of the flow-volume loop can help to distinguish different disease states (Figure 7.3).

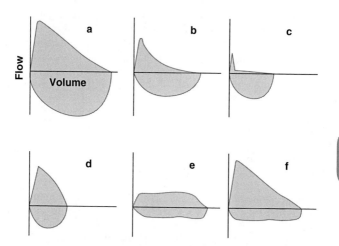

Figure 7.3 The normal flow-volume loop is shown together with examples of how respiratory disease can alter its shape: (a) normal subject; (b) obstructive airway disease (e.g. asthma); (c) severe obstructive disease (e.g. emphysema); (d) restrictive lung disease (e.g. pulmonary fibrosis); (e) fixed major airway obstruction (e.g. carcinoma of the trachea); and (f) floppy extra-thoracic airway obstruction (e.g. tracheomalacia).

However, note that the inspiratory curve is effort-dependent and thus very sensitive to submaximal effort, whereas the expiratory curve is largely independent of effort. Severe emphysema often causes a very rapid decrease in expiratory flow that is dependent on expiratory effort, whereas inspiratory flow is well preserved (Figure 7.3(c)). In emphysema, the airways are prone to rapid collapse and/or narrowing during forced expiration (*pressure-dependent*) due to a loss of elastic tissue airway support with the obliteration of the alveolar walls. During inspiration, the airways are easily dilated, preserving inspiratory flows. If the airflow limitation is due to airways disease (e.g. asthma), the scalloping of the expiratory curve is more gradual and less effort-dependent (*volume-dependent collapse*). The inspiratory flows are also reduced, suggesting that the cause of the airflow limitation is relatively 'fixed'.

Truncation of inspiratory flow may result from a floppy extra-thoracic airway (e.g. tracheomalacia of the larynx, fractured larynx), whereas both inspiratory and expiratory flows are truncated for fixed lesions (e.g. carcinoma of the trachea). Expiratory flows alone may be reduced for intra-thoracic lesions of the large airways (e.g. tracheo-malacia of the lower trachea and main bronchi). Further examples of the different flow-volume loop shapes are given in Figure 7.4.

The flow-volume loop is also useful for assessing ventilatory impairment during exercise. The tidal volume and inspiratory and expiratory flows increase with exercise but *are constrained within the boundary of the maximum flow-volume loop*. In the presence of airflow limitation, the patient's capacity to increase ventilation to meet the body's increased metabolic demands during exercise is limited. This is illustrated in Figure 7.5 where the capacity to exercise will be clearly impaired due to reduced capacity to ventilate—a consequence of the curvilinearity in the maximal expiratory flow-volume curve. Once tidal breathing hits the boundary of the flow-volume curve, the only way to further increase ventilation is for the patient to breathe at a higher lung volume where there is more 'room' to ventilate. In exercise, expiratory time becomes reduced and this tends to increase functional residual capacity (FRC), yet tidal volume is increased so that end-expiratory volume is even further increased compared with its resting or quiet breathing level. The increase in end-expiratory volume (FRC) can be measured as a decrease in inspiratory capacity. Patients with severe airflow obstruction thus develop dynamic hyperinflation during exercise and this expands the envelope of flow rates achievable within the tidal breathing range.

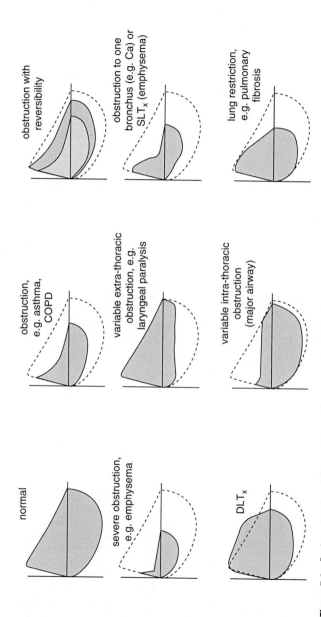

Figure 7.4 Further examples of how respiratory disease can alter the shape of the flow-volume loop.

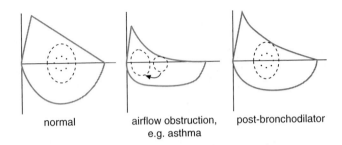

normal   airflow obstruction,   post-bronchodilator
                      e.g. asthma

Figure 7.5 These flow-volume loops illustrate how the boundary of the maximum loop can limit minute ventilation and thereby impede exercise tolerance (see text). The dotted loops represent tidal breathing at rest and during exercise.

Inspiratory capacity (IC) is a measure of the maximum volume that can be inspired from FRC to TLC. The IC is reduced both in obstructive diseases when hyperinflation is present (Figure 7.6) and in restrictive disease when total lung capacity is reduced. When airflow obstruction has been identified by reductions in FEV_1, FVC and FEV_1/FVC, the IC affords a good measure of hyperinflation and is reduced in airways disease because FRC is increased. Hyperinflation may be chronic and stable as in emphysema but may increase with exercise or acute worsening of airflow obstruction. It may improve with bronchodilation or with oxygen therapy, which reduces ventilatory equivalents and permits slower breathing with more time for expirations so that a lower end-expiratory lung volume is achieved.

There is currently much interest in the measurement of IC, both during quiet breathing and developing dynamically during exercise, as a sensitive marker of change and treatment response in COPD because changes in dynamic hyperinflation may occur without much change in maximal expired volumes, for example, FEV_1 and FVC.

Although the measurement of IC in clinical practice requires further evaluation, it may well prove of clinical utility in assessing progress and treatment response in the individual with COPD. Recent research has shown that IC correlates better than FEV_1, FVC and so on, with improvement in dyspnoea, exercise tolerance and quality of life measures in the disease.

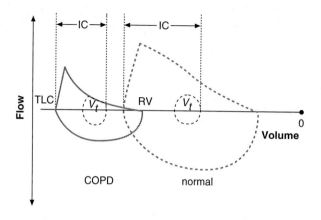

Figure 7.6 Flow-volume curve from a patient with COPD (predicted curve is dotted), showing displacement to the left (hyperinflation), limited tidal flows and reduced inspiratory capacity.

GRADING SEVERITY OF A VENTILATORY DEFECT

There are currently no universally accepted criteria for grading the severity of ventilatory defects. However, FEV_1 expressed as a percentage of the mean predicted value is usually used to grade the severity of obstructive defects because it usually correlates with the severity of symptoms and prognosis. Grading the severity of *any* spirometric impairment (obstructive, restrictive and mixed defects) based on the $FEV_1\%$ predicted has been recommended by the ATS/ERS (Pellegrino et al. 2005) and is given in Table 7.3. Note that in patients with upper airway obstruction (e.g. tracheal stenosis) the use of $FEV_1\%$ predicted to grade the severity of an obstructive defect may result in underestimation of severity and is not recommended (Pellegrino et al. 2005). The use of the FEV_1/FVC ratio to grade obstruction is not generally recommended because obstructive lung disease can reduce both FEV_1 and FVC and also the ratio does not provide any information about the absolute values that determine the capacity to ventilate and degree of respiratory impairment. A reduced $FEF_{25-75\%}$ in the presence of a normal FEV_1, FVC and FEV_1/FVC is usually regarded as an indication of a mild obstructive defect.

TABLE 7.3	Grading the severity of a spirometric impairment
FEV$_1$ % predicted	**Severity grading**
> 70	Mild obstructive defect
60–69	Moderate obstructive defect
50–59	Moderately severe obstructive defect
35–49	Severe obstructive defect
< 35	Very severe obstructive defect

Source: Pellegrino et al. (2005).

MEASURING REVERSIBILITY OF AIRFLOW OBSTRUCTION

To measure the degree of reversibility (typically increased in asthma) of airflow obstruction, perform spirometry before and 10 to 15 minutes after administering a bronchodilator by metered dose inhaler or jet nebuliser. Short-acting β-agonists (e.g. albutamol/salbutamol or terbutaline) are generally considered the benchmark bronchodilators for reversibility testing. If slower-acting agents (such as ipratropium bromide) are used, the post-bronchodilator test should be conducted at least 30 minutes after its administration.

FEV$_1$ is the most common index used to quantify the degree of improvement. To determine the degree of improvement, calculate the following:

- the *absolute change* in FEV$_1$ (post-bronchodilator FEV$_1$ minus baseline FEV$_1$), and
- the *percentage increase* from the baseline FEV$_1$:

$$\% \text{ improvement} = 100 \times \frac{\text{FEV}_1 \text{ (post-bronchodilator)} - \text{FEV}_1 \text{ (baseline)}}{\text{FEV}_1 \text{ (baseline)}}$$

There is presently no universal agreement on the definition of significant bronchodilator reversibility. According to the ATS/ERS, the criteria for a positive response in adults are (Pellegrino et al. 2005):

Increase in FEV$_1$ (and/or FVC) from baseline ≥ 12% and ≥ 0.2 L.

If possible the patient should not use their short-acting bronchodilator (e.g. albutamol/salbutamol, ipratropium bromide) within four hours of testing. Long-acting inhaled bronchodilators (e.g. salmeterol) should be withheld for 12 hours prior to reversibility testing.

The most common method for administering the inhaled bronchodilator for reversibility testing is via a valved spacer. When albutamol/salbutamol is used it is common to administer four separate doses of 100 µg (total 400 µg), allowing a 30-second interval between each dose.

Normal subjects generally exhibit a smaller degree of reversibility (up to 8% in most studies). The absence of reversibility does not exclude asthma because an asthmatic's response can vary from time to time and at times airway calibre in asthmatic subjects is clearly normal and incapable of dramatic improvement.

Bronchodilator response based on an improvement in $FEF_{25-75\%}$ can be difficult to interpret as it varies with FVC, which is often larger post-bronchodilator. Thus, it is not recommended that $FEF_{25-75\%}$ be used to assess reversibility. Assessment of improvement in IC post-broncho-dilator (often paralleling improvement in symptoms), indicating a decreased degree of hyperinflation, may indicate a significant response even when FEV_1 is unchanged in patients with COPD. However, not all office spirometers measure IC. This illustrates the complexity of assessing bronchodilator response and that reliance on the change in FEV_1 (or FVC) alone can be inadequate and should not necessarily preclude prescribing a bronchodilator on a trial basis. This measurement of IC is not commonly made in general practice at present but may be of clinical value and become more utilised in the future.

Accurate and reproducible measurements can be influenced by the amount of bronchodilator delivered to the airways. Studies have demonstrated that a reduced amount of bronchodilator to the airways can result in less than maximal bronchodilator improvement. As a result, patients tested would not demonstrate the optimal result that the bronchodilator could deliver.

If a metered dose inhaler is to be used, carefully check the subject's inhaler technique. About 30% of adults and 50% of children do not use their metered dose inhalers correctly. If incorrect use occurs, the use of a valved spacer device or jet nebuliser to improve aerosol delivery would be appropriate.

AIRWAY PROVOCATION TESTING

The measurement of airway hyperresponsiveness is rarely performed in a doctor's surgery and will not be discussed in detail.

The airway provocation test is used to detect and quantify airway hyperreactivity, an important feature of clinical asthma; quantitatively, airway hyperresponsiveness is thought to reflect asthma severity. However, some asthmatics may have a negative challenge, particularly if being treated with corticosteroids, and normal subjects with no history of asthma or variability in spirometry may return positive challenge results, particularly following recent upper respiratory tract infection.

In this test the patient is exposed to a stimulus that may induce bronchospasm, such as:

- exercise
- isocapnic hyperventilation
- hypertonic saline aerosol
- methacholine aerosol
- histamine aerosol
- mannitol aerosol.

The test involves measuring FEV_1 at baseline and then at intervals following the stimuli. Unlike measuring bronchodilator response, here the effect of the stimulus is to decrease ventilatory function. The most common bronchial provocation agent is methacholine, which is delivered to the airway as an aerosol and stimulates cholinergic receptors in airway smooth muscle. Progressively increasing doses of methacholine are administered with measurements of FEV_1 between each dose. The test is positive and terminated when the FEV_1 falls by 20% from the baseline value (called the provoking dose, $PD_{20\%}$—see Figure 7.7). A positive response indicates heightened airway reactivity

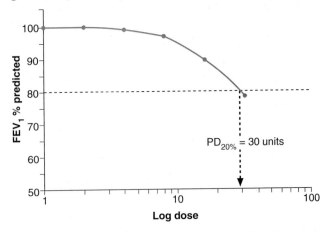

Figure 7.7 Generalised plot of FEV_1 versus provoking dose. The test is terminated when the FEV_1 falls by 20% from the baseline value; the concentration or dose of agent causing this degree of fall is reported as the $PD_{20\%}$.

(airway narrowing in response to the stimulus). Treatment with anti-inflammatory agents is designed to suppress bronchial reactivity in patients with asthma, resulting in an increase in the dose of provoking agent necessary to reduce the FEV_1.

PEAK FLOW MONITORING

The availability of inexpensive peak flow meters and pocket spirometers has allowed the physician to directly involve patients in the management of their disease by self-monitoring airway function. This is particularly so in asthma, where regular peak flow monitoring is commonly part of a written management plan negotiated between the patient and his or her doctor. It is also particularly useful for the assessment of occupational asthma, where PEF readings performed at work are compared with baseline readings recorded during periods off work and may reveal a clear relationship between work exposure and bronchoconstriction, with recovery on weekends, holidays and so on, or with treatment. A typical record is given in Figure 7.8.

Measurement of PEF is simpler than spirometry. Its limitations are that it is effort-dependent, insensitive to obstructions of small and peripheral airways, and that the inter- and intra-subject variability is

Figure 7.8 Self-monitoring of PEF over seven days for a worker who attends work Monday to Friday with weekends off. Note that the PEF increases at the weekends when the worker is not at work.

about twice that of FEV_1. This is particularly true in children where PEF can be unreliable as they are often unable to perform the test with consistent maximal efforts. So diurnal variation, even in healthy children, can be as high as 30%. The physician should provide the patient with clear, written instructions about how to perform and record his or her PEF. It is essential to stress the importance of accurate recordings of PEF and to motivate the patient.

When PEF is measured repeatedly over a period and plotted against time (e.g. by asthmatic patients), the pattern of the graph can be very important in identifying particular aspects of the patient's disease. Typical patterns are:

- the fall in PEF during the week with improvement on weekends and holidays which occurs in occupational asthma (Figure 7.8)
- the 'morning dipper' pattern of some asthmatic patients caused by a fall in PEF in the early morning hours (Figure 7.9). Isolated falls in PEF in relation to specific allergens or trigger factors can help to identify and quantify these for the doctor and patient. A downward trend in PEF and an increase in its variability can identify worsening asthma and can be used to guide therapy. PEF monitoring is particularly useful in the substantial number of asthmatic people with poor perception of their own airway calibre. Response to asthma treatment is usually accompanied by an increase in PEF and a decrease in its variability.

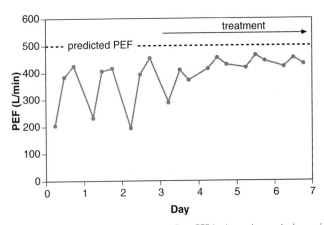

Figure 7.9 The 'morning dipper' pattern (low PEF in the early morning) seen in some asthmatic patients. Note the improvement in the 'dips' with increased anti-inflammatory treatment.

Remember that many patients have poor perception of their own airflow obstruction and their PEF is a better index of the state of their airways than how they feel.

CHOOSING THE APPROPRIATE TEST

It is important to recognise likely clinical situations and to choose the appropriate test for each. For example (see also Chapter 1):

- For patients with respiratory symptoms such as dyspnoea, wheeze, chronic cough and sputum production and exercise intolerance, spirometry and DLCO are indicated to diagnose and differentiate diseases causing ventilatory abnormality of obstructive or restrictive type.
- In patients with COPD, spirometry is indicated to follow the progression of the disease, response to interventions and so on.
- For the diagnosis of asthma, obtain spirometry before and after the administration of a bronchodilator, looking for an obstructive pattern with significant improvement. It is usually necessary to repeat spirometry at follow-up visits in asthma and other lung conditions where change can occur over short periods of time.
- In patients suspected of having asthma but in whom baseline spirometry is normal, it may be appropriate to confirm the diagnosis by measuring airway reactivity by provocation testing, with measurement of spirometry before and after provocation by exercise or by inhalation of methacholine or mannitol.
- To identify asthma triggers or treatment responses over long periods of time, regular PEF monitoring by the asthmatic patient is more reliable than a symptom diary alone.
- If upper airway obstruction is suspected, flow-volume loop with particular emphasis on inspiration is the best test.
- To assess the risk of postoperative complications in the elderly and respiratory compromised, particularly if undergoing abdominal or thoracic surgery, the FEV_1, FVC and FEV_1/FVC ratio are the most useful indices. If an obstructive ventilatory defect is present, the anaesthetist would like to know whether there was improvement after administration of a bronchodilator.
- To assess smoking-related damage, evidence of airflow obstruction should be sought systematically using spirometry. This information may be helpful in convincing smokers to give up the habit.

Serial spirometric measurements are useful to quantify severity and to follow the progression and response to therapy of respiratory diseases such as COPD, asthma and interstitial lung disease. Here measures such as FEV_1 and FVC may be helpful in asthma, but in COPD measurement of IC as an index of functional hyperinflation also has clinical utility and better correlation with functional outcomes (O'Donnell 2000). Although detailed studies are needed to better establish the magnitude of a clinically meaningful change, an increase of about 10% in dynamic IC with exercise may be considered a clinically significant improvement. Such increases correlate with dyspnoea scores and exercise endurance time.

SUMMARY

Abnormal spirometry is usually classified as an obstructive, restrictive or mixed ventilatory defect. The most commonly seen defect is airflow obstruction, which is characterised by reduced expiratory flows (e.g. COPD and current asthma) and usually results in a curvilinear expiratory flow-volume curve. In a restrictive ventilatory defect the patient has no difficulty blowing out quickly, but the FVC (and VC) are significantly reduced due to small lungs (e.g. pulmonary fibrosis). A mixed ventilatory defect is characterised by both airflow obstruction and small lungs. The shape of the flow-volume loop can be useful diagnostically and can be interpreted at a glance. The degree of reversibility of airflow obstruction following the administration of a bronchodilator is commonly assessed. A significant response is considered to have occurred if the FEV_1 (or FVC) improves by $\geq$ 12% and $\geq$ 0.2 litre compared to pre-bronchodilator values. The degree of airway hyperresponsiveness can be assessed by measuring spirometry before and after incremental doses of a bronchoconstricting agent or exercise.

CHAPTER 8

CASE HISTORIES

The cases histories in this section illustrate the utility of spirometry in the diagnosis and management of patients with lung disease or respiratory symptoms and in the screening of subjects (e.g. pre-employment, scuba diving and preoperative screening).

The mean predicted and lower limit of normal (LLN) are given; the latter is used to determine whether a given result is abnormal and the former is used to compute the per cent predicted.

Note that the interpretation of spirometry is greatly facilitated when the patient's symptoms (e.g. wheezing), smoking history, breathlessness on exertion, recent bronchodilator use and the clinical questions being asked are known. Interpretation is also facilitated by estimating the pre-test probability of lung disease. For example, a patient with a significant smoking history, breathlessness on exertion and wheeze would have a high pre-test probability of chronic obstructive pulmonary disease (COPD).

Note that in the following cases the identification of an apparent restrictive defect on spirometry needs to be confirmed and quantified by measuring lung volumes.

CASE 1

Case history

- Male aged 25 years
- Never smoked
- No history of respiratory disease
- Normal chest X-ray
- Referred for pre-employment lung function tests

Results

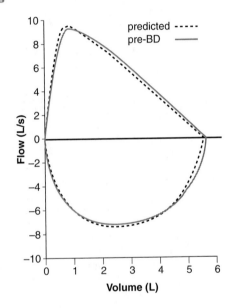

	Predicted mean (LLN)	Pre-BD	Post-BD
FEV_1 (L)	4.44 (3.67)	4.35	–
FVC (L)	5.36 (4.46)	5.60	–
FEV_1/FVC	0.83 (0.73)	0.78	–
$FEF_{25-75\%}$ (L/s)	4.6 (3.1)	5.3	–
PEF (L/s)	10.0 (7.7)	9.8	–

Technical comment: Test performance was good.

Interpretation

The shape of the flow-volume loop and all spirometric indices are within the normal range, indicating normal ventilatory function. This provides useful baseline lung function data for future comparison.

8

CASE 2

Case history

- Male aged 20 years
- Smoked since age 15
- History of episodic wheeze and chest tightness, particularly in the early morning and during exercise. PEF performed by his family doctor was 43% of the predicted value
- Referred for possible asthma

Results

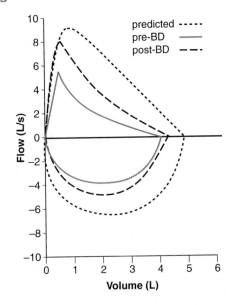

	Predicted mean (LLN)	Pre-BD	Post-BD
FEV$_1$ (L)	4.30 (3.58)	2.25	3.20
FVC (L)	5.10 (4.25)	4.25	4.40
FEV$_1$/FVC	0.83 (0.74)	0.53	0.73
FEF$_{25-75\%}$ (L/s)	4.7 (3.2)	2.1	3.9
PEF (L/s)	9.4 (7.3)	5.5	8.3

Technical comment: Test performance was good.

Interpretation

The concavity in the expiratory flow-volume curve indicates an obstructive ventilatory defect. Pre-bronchodilator FEV_1/FVC ratio is 0.53 and FEV_1 is 52% predicted, indicating a moderately severe obstructive ventilatory defect. There was a 42% (0.95 L) improvement in FEV_1 post-bronchodilator indicating substantial reversibility.

Pathophysiology: These results are highly suggestive of asthma. In asthma, the airflow obstruction is due to contraction of bronchial smooth muscle (reversible), inflammatory thickening of bronchial mucosa (may improve with steroids) and mucus in the bronchial tubes. Hyperinflation may be present (high TLC and/or FRC), but the diffusing capacity of the lung for carbon monoxide (DLCO) is normal.

8

CASE 3

Case history

- Male aged 73 years
- Smoker of 50 years (65 pack-years)
- History of increasing shortness of breath, chest infections, chronic cough and hospital admissions (twice in the past two years) for respiratory failure secondary to pneumonia
- Recent chest X-ray shows flat diaphragms and hyperlucent lungs
- Referred for lung function tests to document ventilatory function and response to bronchodilator

Results

	Predicted mean (LLN)	Pre-BD	Post-BD
FEV_1 (L)	2.54 (1.84)	0.85	0.90
FVC (L)	3.81 (3.10)	2.10	2.20
FEV_1/FVC	0.82 (0.73)	0.40	0.41
$FEF_{25-75\%}$ (L/s)	3.2 (1.9)	0.9	0.9
PEF (L/s)	7.1 (5.4)	3.6	3.6

Technical comment: Test performance was acceptable.

Interpretation

The deep concavity in the expiratory flow-volume curve and low FEV_1/FVC ratio and low FEV_1 (33% predicted) indicate a very severe obstructive ventilatory defect. There was no significant improvement post-bronchodilator (salbutamol plus ipratropium bromide). These results are consistent with severe COPD.

Pathophysiology: In COPD, the airflow obstruction is due to inflammatory thickening and distortion of the airway walls (small airway disease) and to expiratory collapse of airways due to loss of elastic support (emphysema) from the parenchyma. The VC is often well preserved until the disease is severe. In emphysema RV, FRC and TLC are usually increased, indicating gas trapping (high RV) and hyperinflation (high FRC and/or TLC). The DLCO is also reduced.

8

CASE 4

Case history

- Female aged 40 years, BMI 35
- Ex-smoker for 10 years
- Chronic cough
- No significant history of respiratory disease other than occasional upper respiratory tract infections
- No unusual findings on recent chest X-ray
- Referred for routine lung function tests prior to a cholecystectomy

Results

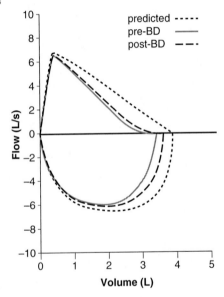

	Predicted mean (LLN)	Pre-BD	Post-BD
FEV_1 (L)	3.11 (2.51)	2.59	2.68
FVC (L)	3.81 (3.10)	3.35	3.45
FEV_1/FVC	0.82 (0.73)	0.75	0.77
$FEF_{25-75\%}$ (L/s)	3.2 (1.9)	1.6	1.8
PEF (L/s)	7.1 (5.4)	6.9	6.9

Technical comment: Performance of test was good.

Interpretation

The expiratory flow-volume curve shows abnormally low flows at low lung volumes (and low $FEF_{25-75\%}$) suggesting that the small airways rather than the large airways are abnormally narrow during forced expiration. This is confirmed by the normal FEV_1 and PEF but reduced $FEF_{25-75\%}$ (less than the LLN). Post-bronchodilator, there was no significant improvement in FEV_1 or small airway function. These results suggest the presence of small airway disease, probably the result of her smoking history, although mild asthma is not ruled out. There is probably no increased risk of postoperative pulmonary complications.

CASE 5

Case history

- Male aged 40 years
- Recent history of waking early in the morning with chest tightness and cough
- The general practitioner (GP) gave him a peak flow meter to monitor his PEF on waking, at noon and before retiring
- After reviewing the results, the physician prescribed salbutamol prn and inhaled steroids bid.
- The patient then monitored his PEF again for a week and then again 30 days later.

Results

Pre-treatment

Patient on asthma therapy

Interpretation

The pre-treatment peak flow chart collected over a seven-day period shows wide swings in PEF (195 to 440 L/min) with the lowest readings occurring in the morning upon waking. During the day, the PEF increased to near the predicted value. These results support the patient's symptoms and are diagnostic of asthma. The GP prescribed salbutamol and inhaled corticosteroids. A further seven days of self-monitoring showed marked improvement in PEF and the patient's symptoms resolved.

Pathophysiology: These results are highly suggestive of asthma. In asthma, the airflow obstruction is due to contraction of bronchial smooth muscle (reversible), inflammatory thickening of bronchial mucosa and mucus in the bronchial tubes.

8

CASE 6

Case history

- Female of 40 years
- Non-smoker, no past history of respiratory problems
- Five years of joint aches and morning stiffness; dyspnoea for past three months
- Recent chest X-ray shows diffuse lung filtrate
- Referred for assessment of dyspnoea

Results

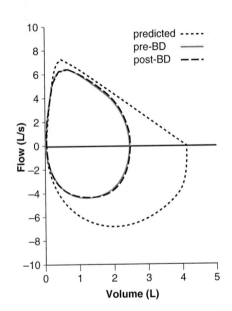

	Predicted mean (LLN)	Pre-BD	Post-BD
FEV_1 (L)	3.30 (2.66)	2.21	2.25
FVC (L)	4.06 (3.31)	2.45	2.50
FEV_1/FVC	0.82 (73)	0.90	0.90
$FEF_{25-75\%}$ (L/s)	3.3 (2.0)	4.1	4.3
PEF (L/s)	7.4 (5.6)	6.3	6.4

Technical comment: Test performance was good.

Interpretation

The flow-volume loop shows a reduced FVC and FEV_1 with a well-preserved FEV_1/FVC ratio and maximal flows. This is consistent with a restrictive ventilatory defect. FVC is 60% predicted so this is a moderate restrictive defect. As expected, there is no significant change after bronchodilator.

Pathophysiology: In this patient, the restrictive ventilatory defect was found to be due to fibrosing alveolitis associated with rheumatoid arthritis. The expiratory flows are well preserved relative to her reduced lung volume (TLC was 67% predicted) due to increased traction on the airways from the stiff parenchymal tissue. The static lung volumes (TLC, FRC, RV) are reduced because the overall size of the lungs is restricted by inflammatory and fibrotic scar tissue. The DLCO is reduced due to inflammation and fibrosis of the alveolar–capillary membrane.

Successful therapy of her RA with prednisolone was associated with improved FVC and DLCO.

8

CASE 7

Case history

- Male aged 30 years
- Non-smoker, no past history of respiratory problems
- Presents with two years of progressive limb muscle weakness and wasting
- In the past two months has noted exertional breathlessness and mild daytime sleepiness
- Recent chest X-ray is normal
- Referred for investigation of his increased breathlessness

Results

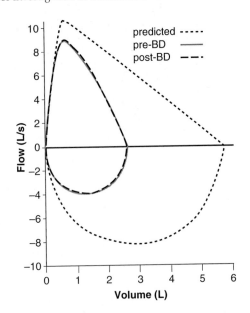

	Predicted mean (LLN)	Pre-BD	Post-BD
FEV$_1$ (L)	4.58 (3.77)	1.90	1.95
FVC (L)	5.62 (4.67)	2.35	2.35
FEV$_1$/FVC	0.82 (0.72)	0.81	0.83
FEF$_{25-75\%}$ (L/s)	4.6 (2.9)	6.2	6.2
PEF (L/s)	10.5 (8.1)	8.9	9.2

Technical comment: Test performance was fairly good.

Interpretation

The flow-volume loop shows normal expiratory but reduced inspiratory flows consistent with weak inspiratory muscles (diaphragm). The FVC is markedly reduced (42% predicted), suggesting a severe restrictive ventilatory defect. Further investigation showed that the maximal inspiratory pressure that the patient can generate is only 30 cmH$_2$O and daytime hypercapnoea is present. These results are consistent with diaphragmatic weakness as part of a muscular dystrophy. The nocturnal daytime sleepiness is probably due to sleep fragmentation associated with nocturnal worsening of respiratory failure during sleep. The DLCO is usually within normal limits.

8

CASE 8

Case history

- Male aged 65 years
- Long history of cigarette smoking (50 pack-years)
- Gradually increasing cough, breathlessness, and sputum has recently been tinged with blood
- Recent chest X-ray shows thickening of the mediastinum and right upper lobe mass
- Spirometry is requested pre-bronchoscopy

Results

	Predicted mean (LLN)	Pre-BD	Post-BD
FEV_1 (L)	3.50 (2.70)	2.20	2.30
FVC (L)	4.69 (3.75)	4.10	4.15
FEV_1/FVC	0.75 (0.65)	0.54	0.55
$FEF_{25-75\%}$ (L/s)	2.8 (1.2)	2.1	2.3
PEF (L/s)	8.9 (6.6)	4.4	4.5

Technical comment: This patient had difficulty following instructions due to a hearing impairment. However, the patient eventually responded to visual prompts and was able to produce acceptable and repeatable forced manoeuvres.

Interpretation

An obstructive ventilatory defect (low FEV_1/FVC ratio) with little improvement post-bronchodilator. The flow-volume loop shows a plateau in both expiratory and inspiratory flows (i.e. truncation). The FVC is little affected but it takes a longer time than normal to empty, as indicated by the reduced FEV_1/FVC ratio. The shape of the flow-volume loop is characteristic of a rigid large airway obstruction. In this case, the cause is an obstructing carcinoma of the trachea.

CASE 9

Case history

- Male aged 30 years
- Injured in a football match with an accidental kick to the throat when knocked down in a crowded pack
- Struggled for breath when carried from the ground by trainers
- Noted to have marked inspiratory stridor and agitation when brought to casualty by ambulance
- Spirometry was performed with difficulty in casualty

Results

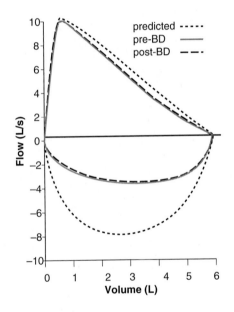

	Predicted mean (LLN)	Pre-BD	Post-BD
FEV_1 (L)	4.83 (3.98)	4.75	4.70
FVC (L)	5.96 (4.96)	5.95	5.80
FEV_1/FVC	0.82 (0.72)	0.80	0.81
$FEF_{25-75\%}$ (L/s)	4.7 (3.0)	4.5	4.5
PEF (L/s)	10.9 (8.4)	10.7	10.8

Technical comment: Test performance was only fair.

Interpretation

The major abnormality in the flow-volume loop is selective truncation of maximal inspiratory flow. This is caused during inspiration by the extra-thoracic upper airway collapsing as it has lost its rigid support and is sucked inward by a negative intra-luminal pressure (i.e. subatmospheric pressure). The maximal expiratory flow is normal as a positive intra-luminal pressure is developed, causing the upper airway to distend. The shape of this flow-volume loop is typical of a floppy (i.e. dynamic) extra-thoracic airway obstruction. In this case, the cause was a fractured larynx.

8

CASE 10

Case history

- Female aged 45 years
- Long history of smoking (35 pack-years)
- Recent history of chest tightness, especially on the left side
- Weight loss is starting to occur
- Chest X-ray is within normal limits
- Spirometry is requested, as is a bronchoscopy

Results

	Predicted mean (LLN)	Pre-BD	Post-BD
FEV$_1$ (L)	2.64 (2.11)	1.35	1.40
FVC (L)	3.27 (2.64)	2.45	2.45
FEV$_1$/FVC	0.81 (0.72)	0.55	0.57
FEF$_{25-75\%}$ (L/s)	2.8 (1.7)	1.3	1.4
PEF (L/s)	6.4 (4.9)	3.1	3.0

Technical comment: Test performance was good.

Interpretation

An obstructive ventilatory defect is present (low FEV_1 and FEV_1/FVC ratio, and curvilinearity in descending limb of the expiratory flow-volume curve) with little reversibility post-bronchodilator. The FEV_1 is 51% predicted indicating that the obstructive defect is moderately severe. The shape of the flow-volume loop is an unusual biconcave with marked flow reduction in the latter parts of both the inspiratory and expiratory curves. This shape is consistent with carcinoma of one of the main bronchi. Since one bronus is obstructed, air flows at unequal rates from the left and right lungs. In this patient, the right lung empties and fills much faster than the left (obstructed) lung.

CASE 11

Case history

- Male aged 45 years
- Current smoker (16 pack-years) with chronic productive cough and breathlessness on exertion
- COPD was suspected and spirometry performed as part of the clinical assessment of COPD

Results

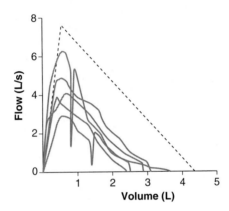

Technical comment: Test performance was very variable due to submaximal effort. Test terminated at request of patient.

Interpretation

This is an example of a subject performing spirometry with variable effort. Both the start-of-test (back-extrapolated volume) and end-of-test criteria (plateau) were not met, and there was evidence of cough artifact and failure to commence the forced expiration at full inspiration. The results cannot reliably be compared with predicted values or used to monitor serial changes or response to therapy.

SUMMARY

These case histories demonstrate the value of measuring spirometry in clinical practice. The most common abnormalities are intermittent and chronic airflow obstruction characterised by reduced expiratory flows. In addition, serial measurements can be very useful in the management of patients to assess intermittent airways obstruction, disease progression and response to therapy. The cases also illustrate the value of the shape of the flow-volume curve or loop in the interpretation of results. Several of the cases (especially Case 9) illustrate the importance of recording the inspired as well as expired flow-volume curve. In Case 9, expiration is normal and the life-threatening abnormality would have been missed using equipment that did not report inspiration. However, the results obtained are of clinical value only if the test is performed using a calibrated spirometer and the patient has been actively coaxed to perform the correct breathing manoeuvre (Case 11).

CHAPTER 9

MECHANICS OF BREATHING

GAS FLOW THROUGH THE AIRWAYS—HOW AIRFLOW IS PRODUCED

Gas will flow through any tube if the pressure at one end is higher than that at the other. The magnitude of the gas flow will depend largely on the pressure difference between the ends of the tube and the resistance of the tube. The latter has components of frictional resistance between the gas molecules and the side wall of the tube and the energy required to produce convective acceleration of the gas molecules.

In life, the respiratory muscles generate pressure in the pleural space surrounding the lung that, in turn, influences alveolar pressure (the pressure driving gas in and out of the lung). The pressure difference between the alveoli and lips ($P_1 - P_2$), produces airflow and the magnitude of the airflow depends on the resistance of the airways, according to the relationship shown in Figure 9.1.

$$\text{flow} = \frac{P_1 - P_2}{\text{resistance}}$$

Figure 9.1 Factors determining flow of gas through an airway.

Tidal breathing

Inspiratory work is performed by the diaphragm and intercostal muscles to generate a negative pressure within the pleural space. This creates a negative alveolar pressure that results in inspiratory airflow. Normally, expiration at rest is a passive process with expiratory flow produced by the potential energy stored in the elastic lung tissue with relaxation of the inspiratory muscles. During quiet breathing in healthy subjects, the pressure in the pleural space (P_{pl}) is about 4 or 5 cmH$_2$O below atmospheric during inspiration and 4 or 5 cmH$_2$O above atmospheric during expiration.

Forced respiratory manoeuvres

The respiratory muscles generate large intra-pleural pressures, and both forced inspiration and forced expiration are active processes. The large pleural pressure creates a much larger pressure difference between the alveoli and lips, thus producing a much greater airflow than during quiet breathing.

PATTERNS OF AIRFLOW IN THE HUMAN AIRWAYS

The human bronchial tree consists of some 26 generations of branching tubes from the single trachea to the very numerous terminal bronchioles. Figure 9.2 shows that the total cross-sectional area of the airways increases greatly from a few square centimetres in the trachea to a total area of about 10 000 square centimetres at the level of the last generation of terminal bronchioles.

This means that the speed gas moves through the tracheobronchial tree will vary greatly. In the trachea and main bronchi, the gas velocity will be high (small cross-sectional area) but it will travel very slowly through the peripheral airways (large cross-sectional area).

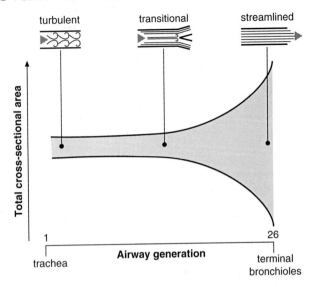

Figure 9.2 Flow profiles during forced expiration. In the large airways where cross-sectional area is small, flow is turbulent. Peripherally where cross-sectional area is large, flow is streamlined (or laminar). In between, particularly at branch points, flow is transitional.

The large differences in gas velocity affect the pattern of gas flow in different parts of the tracheobronchial tree (Figure 9.2). In the peripheral airways where gas velocity is low, a *streamlined* (or laminar) flow pattern is present, whereas in the trachea, where gas velocity is relatively high, the flow pattern is *turbulent*. In the medium-sized airways, the flow pattern is a mixture of streamlined and turbulent and is termed *transitional*.

The relevance of these different flow patterns is that they vary in the efficiency with which the pressure difference (or energy) is expended in producing gas flow. The flow patterns are also affected by the physical properties of the gas (such as gas density).

Under *streamlined* flow conditions, flow is directly proportional to the pressure drop along the airways and is described by Poiseuille's equation:

$$\text{Flow} = (P_1 - P_2) \times \frac{\pi \times r^4}{\mu \times 8 \times L}$$

$$\text{Thus airway resistance} = \frac{(P_1 - P_2)}{\text{Flow}} = \frac{\mu \times 8 \times L}{\pi \times r^4}$$

where $(P_1 - P_2)$ is the pressure drop along the airways when a gas of viscosity μ flows at a given volume rate. L and r are the length and radius of the airway respectively. This pattern is efficient in terms of pressure expenditure. Note that streamline flow is independent of gas density but is dependent on gas viscosity. Also note that flow and airway resistance are very sensitive to airway radius; if r is doubled, airway resistance decreases 16-fold and if r is halved, $(P_1 - P_2)$ must increase 16-fold if flow is to remain unchanged.

Under *turbulent* conditions, a much higher pressure is required to produce a given flow:

$$\text{flow} \propto (P_1 - P_2)^2$$

Thus turbulent flow is inefficient in terms of the pressure drop required to produce a given flow. The density of the gas, as well as its viscosity, affects turbulent flow.

THE PHENOMENON OF MAXIMAL AIRFLOW LIMITATION

One might expect that the harder one tries to breathe, the greater the airflow that can be achieved. While this concept applies during maximal inspiration, it is not true during forced expiration. This is demonstrated by constructing *isovolume pressure-flow curves* (Figure 9.3). These curves express the relationship between expired flow and pleural pressure (P_{pl}, an index of expiratory effort generated by expiratory muscles) at varying degrees of expiratory effort. The flow corresponding to pleural pressure is plotted for given lung volumes (e.g. 60%, 70% of the VC). The curve (Figure 9.3) representing near full inspiration (i.e. > 85% VC) shows that the maximum expired flow (PEF for this curve) increases with increasing effort (i.e. P_{pl}). It demonstrates that PEF remains effort-dependent. At lower lung volumes, expiratory flow increases with effort until a flow maximum is reached. Any further increase in effort does not result in further increases in expiratory flow (flow is effort-independent). Here any increase in expiratory effort is offset by an increase in airway resistance due to greater airway compression.

Figure 9.3 Isovolume pressure-flow curve at several lung volumes as a percentage of vital capacity in a normal subject. Expired flow is plotted against pleural pressure. Flow reaches a maximum value at a specific pleural pressure and lung volume; that is, flow does not increase despite increased pleural pressure (effort).

Thus, at high lung volumes maximal expiratory flow becomes independent of effort. This can be seen more easily if we plot both pleural pressure and maximal flow against lung volume during forced inspiration and expiration (see Figure 9.4). As you can see, maximal flow follows pleural pressure (P_{pl}) during inspiration, but during expiration maximal flow falls off independent of pleural pressure.

Maximal inspiratory flow is effort-dependent and is determined by three factors:

1. the effort applied by the patient
2. the strength of the inspiratory muscles
3. the patency of the upper airways which are under a compressive force during inspiration (i.e. subatmospheric pressure inside the airways and atmospheric pressure outside) and will tend to collapse. These airways are supported by the cartilage in the wall of the trachea and the larynx, and the rigidity of these structures is important in maintaining inspiratory flow. There is also an increase in tone in the dilator muscles of the larynx and pharynx;

for example, genioglossus and tensor palatini for the pharynx and the posterior cricopharyngeus cricoarytenoid muscles of the larynx (abductors of vocal folds), just preceding and during inspiration, again stabilising these parts of the upper airway against inspiratory collapse.

A number of theories attempt to explain why maximal expiratory flow is effort-independent. These theories include (1) the equal pressure point, (2) flow-limiting segments developing within the airways and (3) wave-speed theory. These will be outlined briefly as we explore the forces and mechanisms limiting maximal expiratory flow through the airways.

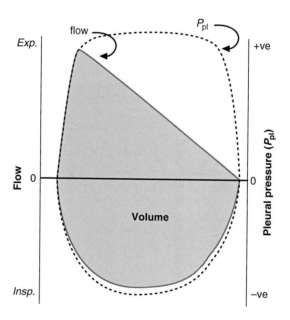

Figure 9.4 Plot of both pleural pressure and maximal flow against volume. Note how the maximal flow follows the degree of effort (P_{pl}) during inspiration but is independent of it during expiration.

THEORIES OF AIRFLOW OBSTRUCTION

The equal pressure point

Imagine if we were to take a snapshot at a particular lung volume during forced expiration and analyse the forces producing expiratory flow (see Figure 9.5). Recall that gas flow from the lung is driven by the pressure difference between the alveoli and the mouth. This pressure difference is dissipated in producing flow so that the pressure at any point inside the airway will be somewhere between alveolar and mouth pressure and will be a distending force during forced expiration.

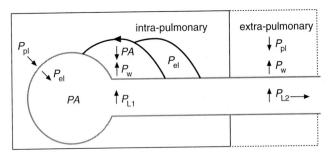

Figure 9.5 Intra-thoracic forces acting on the extra-pulmonary and intra-pulmonary airways. P_{pl} = pleural pressure; P_{el} = elastic recoil pressure; PA = alveolar pressure; P_w = elasticity of the airway wall; P_L = intra-luminal pressure.

The intra-pulmonary airways are surrounded by alveolar pressure that pushes inwards, but they are supported by the elastic recoil of the parenchyma maintained through structural attachments extending to the intra-pulmonary airways and by their own airway wall elasticity (P_w). The pressure acting on the outside wall of the airway (extraluminal pressure) is equal to $PA - P_{el}$ (see Figure 9.5), which we know from analysis of forces on the surface of the lung approximates P_{pl}. Thus, at any instant during expiration the pressure within the alveoli will equal the pleural pressure plus the recoil pressure of the lung (alveolar pressure = $P_{pl} + P_{el}$).

A number of animal studies where the pressure outside the extra-pulmonary airways has been measured during forced expiration have confirmed that this pressure is close to pleural pressure. The pressure across the airway wall (the transmural pressure) will depend on the balance of the pressure outside (pleural pressure) and that inside. Recall that at any point along the airway the pressure will be somewhere between that in the alveoli and at the lips.

The term 'equal pressure point' (EPP) is applied to any point along the airway where the pressure inside the airway equals that outside. Upstream (towards the alveoli during expiration) of the EPP, transmural pressure (P_{tm}) is positive and the airway is distended. However, downstream of the EPP (towards the mouth during expiration) the airway is being compressed because pleural pressure is greater than the pressure within the airway and the elasticity of the airway wall ($P_{pl} > P_{aw}$ and P_{tm} is negative). Because flow is in series, it is possible to describe the maximal expiratory flow (V_{max}) by analysis of the forces in the airway segment upstream from the EPP (R_{us}, resistance of the segment between EPP and alveoli). The driving pressure causing flow (V_{max}) through this segment is the elastic recoil pressure (P_{el}). Thus in the upstream segment:

$$V_{max} = \frac{P_{el}}{R_{us}}$$

Note that the magnitude of the pleural pressure (P_{pl}) does not figure in this equation. Thus, V_{max} depends on the elastic recoil force distending the airways (P_{el}) and the resistance of the airways (R_{us}) and not on pleural pressure (the expiratory effort being generated by the respiratory muscles). Thus, in the downstream segment (between the EPP and mouth):

$$V_{max} = \frac{P_{pl}}{R_{us}}$$

Compression of the airways downstream from the EPP results from greater P_{pl} (i.e. effort) making downstream events more difficult to quantify. However, flow through the upstream segment depends on the static recoil pressure (a fixed property of the lung parenchyma) and the distance of the upstream segment of the airways, which is under distending force and has more constant geometry. It is thus more convenient to describe V_{max} in terms of its upstream components.

Flow-limiting segment

An extension of the EPP theory was put forward by Pride and colleagues in 1967. This group analysed the transmural pressure gradient (P_{tm}) along the airways and led them to conclude that pleural pressure outside the airways downstream of EPP would exceed the pressure within the collapsible airways by a sufficient amount to narrow it 'critically'. This causes flow limitation over a segment of the collapsed downstream airway known as the *flow-limiting segment*. The compliance or elasticity of the downstream airway wall in affecting flow limitation is emphasised in this analysis, which incorporates the EPP concept outlined earlier.

Wave-speed theory

During expiration, pressure waves are propagated in the airway walls from the interaction between the radial recoil force of the elastic walls and the axial inertia of the intraluminal air. The speed of these waves is $(Y\rho)^{0.5}$ where Y (the elastic modulus) is the reciprocal of the specific compliance or distensibility of the airway cross-section and ρ is the density of the gas in the lumen. When airflow through the airway lumen reaches the speed of the pressure wave in the airway wall, flow disturbance causing energy loss prevents any further increase in velocity and a choke point develops at which flow limitation is present.

The flow at *wave speed* (V_{ws}) depends on the cross-sectional area, A, the elasticity of the airway wall ($\delta P_{tm}/\delta A$) and the density ρ of the gas. The maximal flow through the airway is then the product of the speed of these waves and the airway cross-section.

Wave speed through uncompressed airways is high, but downstream of the EPPs a point is reached where the local wave speed reaches a maximal gas velocity and flow limitation occurs. This is referred to as the 'choke point'.

In summary, all these theories are directly applicable and may work in concert during breathing in humans. The current state of our knowledge is that the mechanical properties of the airways (EPP and flow-limiting segment) are responsible for determining V_{max} at low lung volumes. But for high and mid-lung volumes, maximal gas velocity will reach wave speed and flow limitation in large bronchi will occur due to the wave speed rather than effort-related mechanisms. In normal humans, peak expiratory flow during forced expiration occurs very quickly after 25% to 30% of the vital capacity has been expired. Beyond this point, V_{max} becomes independent of effort, provided a certain amount of effort is used. Flow may be then thought of as being determined by:

- elastic recoil pressure of the lung
- flow resistance of the airways between the alveoli and EPP, and
- compliance of the airway wall at choke points.

Consequently, the shape of the maximal expiratory flow-volume curve will depend on changes in either elastic recoil or upstream resistance with volume.

HOW PULMONARY DISEASE AFFECTS AIRFLOW

From the above discussion we have seen how *expiratory flow* is largely independent of effort and relates to the lung elastic recoil pressure, which decreases linearly with lung volume and the resistance of the upstream airways. Maximal *inspiratory flow* on the other hand will depend on the respiratory effort generated, the inspiratory muscle strength and the calibre of the extra-thoracic airway. Disease of the respiratory system influences maximal airflow via a number of mechanisms.

The expired V_{max} will be reduced because of diminished lung elastic recoil in emphysema. However, in asthma and in small airways disease induced by smoking, air pollution and so on, V_{max} will be decreased largely due to increased R_{us} caused by airway wall thickening and narrowing. On the other hand, V_{max} will be well preserved or even increased in interstitial lung disease (e.g. pulmonary fibrosis) where the elastic recoil of the lung tissue is increased and the airways are held wide open by greater than normal elastic recoil forces.

Maximal inspiratory flow is dependent on pleural pressure and airways resistance. Inspiratory flow is thus reduced in asthma and in small airways disease because of the high airways resistance, but is relatively well preserved in emphysema because the airways are distended during inspiration (normal inspiratory airway resistance).

Extra-thoracic airway obstruction (e.g. fractured larynx) is particularly likely to limit inspiratory flow because of compression of the upper airway generated by atmospheric pressure (outside) and low pressure inside the upper airway. Diaphragm weakness limits inspiratory flow through the reduced effort achievable (low P_{pl}). Lack of effort when performing spirometry will also reduce inspiratory flow by the same mechanism.

The above abnormalities result in particular shapes of the flow-volume loops. An understanding of the mechanisms of flow limitation outlined above makes recognition of these specific flow-volume curve shape patterns for specific disease processes a meaningful, rational and reliable diagnostic tool.

9

SUMMARY

Some understanding of the mechanisms of flow limitation greatly assists in the interpretation of spirometry, including the shape of the flow-volume loop. The maximal flow achieved during most of the expiration process is effort-independent because it is determined by the lung's elastic recoil pressure, resistance of the airways between the alveoli and the EPP, and the compliance of the airways at the choke points. During the entire inspiration, maximal flows are effort-dependent.

CHAPTER 10

SUMMARY

Measurements of ventilatory function should be part of the routine assessment of patients with respiratory disease. Spirometry affords clinical practice a simple, achievable, evidence-based and critical opportunity to assess the respiratory health of all who cross its doorstep. It similarly affords the community health practitioner the opportunity to assess the respiratory health of the broader general population. Patient self-monitoring with a peak flow meter or similar device is now an accepted part of the day-to-day management of asthma. Spirometry measurements performed in the lung function laboratory, GP's surgery or respiratory specialist's office can detect and quantify respiratory abnormalities and help to differentiate the various disease processes that result in ventilatory impairment. They also have an important role in following the natural history of respiratory disease and its treatment.

Further, spirometry now has an established place in public health practice as a simple and reliable screening tool for detecting respiratory disease, often before it becomes clinically obvious. The high burden of respiratory disease in the developed world where its roots lie in cigarette smoking, atmospheric pollution and an increasing array of occupational and environmental hazards demands detection and management strategies. People at even higher risk are those in developing countries where indoor combustion practices for cooking and heating remain widespread. Furthermore, spirometry has the capacity to detect airway dysfunction long before symptoms develop, bringing the opportunity to remove harmful exposures before disability develops or becomes severe. These factors render spirometry a critically useful investigation in the detection, management and prevention of respiratory disease.

EQUIPMENT STANDARDS AND VALIDATION PROCEDURES

EQUIPMENT STANDARDS

Those interested in more detailed knowledge of equipment standards and validation procedures are referred to the standardisation document published jointly by the American Thoracic Society and European Respiratory Society (Miller et al. 2005b). This document describes the minimum performance recommendations for all spirometry systems (Table A.1), including monitoring devices, and provides guidelines for their calibration and quality control and gives details of test procedures.

TABLE A.1	Minimum performance recommendations for spirometers

Test	Range/accuracy (BTPS)	Time (s)	Flow range (L/s)	Test signal
VC	0.5 to 8.0 L ±3% of reading or ±0.050 L*	30	0–14	3 L syringe
FVC	0.5 to 8.0 L ±3% of reading or ±0.050 L*	15	0–14	24 ATS waveforms; 3 L syringe
FEV_1	0.5 to 8.0 L ±3% of reading or ±0.050 L*	1	0–14	24 ATS waveforms
Zero time	All timed volumes from a time point determined by back-extrapolation	–	–	Back-extrapolation
PEF	Accuracy: ±10% of reading or ±0.3 L/s* Repeatability: ±5% of reading or ±0.15 L/s*	–	0–14	26 ATS flow waveforms
$FEF_{25-75\%}$	7 L/s ±5% of reading or ±0.2 L/s*	15	±14	24 ATS waveforms
Flow	±14 L/s ±5% of reading or ±0.2 L/s*	15	0–14	Manufacturer's proof

Note: Resistance of entire breathing circuit (including barrier filter, if included) should be less than 1.5 cm H_2O/L/s (0.15 kPa/L/s) over the flow range 0 to 14 L/s for all indices other than PEF. For PEF the resistance at 200, 400 and 600 L/min must be less than 2.5 cm H_2O/L/s (0.25 kPa/L/s).

* Whichever is greater

Source: Miller et al. (2005b).

VALIDATION PROCEDURES

The ATS/ERS also describes *validation procedures* and test signals to assess the accuracy and reproducibility of both volume-displacement and flow spirometers. This requires the use of an expensive computer-controlled syringe that can produce a variety of expiratory FVC curves with accurately known values for FVC, FEV_1, $FEF_{25-75\%}$ and PEF. Validation is normally carried out by the manufacturer (or an independent testing laboratory), and it is important for prospective purchasers to ensure that the spirometer meets the ATS/ERS criteria and that clear documentation of this is provided. Ask for the results before buying a spirometer.

CORRECTION OF VOLUME AND FLOW TO BTPS

For most instruments, manual correction of measured volumes and flows to body temperature and pressure saturated with water vapour (BTPS) is usually necessary when these are calculated from conventional spirograms, as the expired gas contracts due to gas cooling and the condensation of water vapour (Figure B.1). The appropriate correction factor to apply depends on the temperature and to a far

When we blow into a 'cold' spirometer, the volume recorded by the spirometer is less than that displaced from the lungs, due to:
1. gas shrinkage
2. condensation of water vapour (vapour pressure falls)

Figure B.1 Respired volumes (e.g. FEV_1, FVC) and flows (e.g. $FEF_{25-75\%}$) are always corrected to body conditions (BTPS—37°C, fully saturated with water vapour). In this schematic, 2.0 litres are emptied from the lung (BTPS) but only 1.8 litres are recorded by the spirometer (ATPS—ambient temperature and pressure saturated).

lesser extent on the pressure of the gas as it enters the spirometer or flows through the sensor. This correction assumes that expired air cools instantly as it enters the spirometer. Failure to correct values to BTPS can lead to errors of up to 10% in volumes and flows.

Computerised spirometers will usually automatically correct to BTPS, but the operator will need to specify ambient temperature and barometric pressure unless these are measured directly by the instrument.

Heated pneumotachographs partially overcome the need for the temperature correction by reheating expired gas to a temperature close to that of the body, but some further correction may still be required as the gas will have lost water vapour and will not be fully saturated.

The equation for correcting volumes and flow (e.g. FEV_1, $FEF_{25-75\%}$, VC, FVC and PEF) from ATPS to BTPS (assuming expired gas cools instantly to spirometer temperature) is:

$$\text{volume (BTPS)} = \text{volume (ATPS)} \times \frac{P_b - H_2O_t}{P_b - 47} \times \frac{310}{273 + t}$$

Where:

$\quad$ volume (ATPS) = volume measured from spirometer chart

$\qquad\qquad\quad P_b$ = barometric pressure (mmHg)

$\qquad\qquad H_2O_t$ = saturated water vapour pressure (mmHg) at spirometer temperature, t—see Table B.1

$\qquad\qquad\qquad t$ = spirometry temperature (usually equal to room temperature) in degrees Celsius

$\qquad\qquad\quad 47$ = saturated water vapour pressure (mmHg) at $37°C$

Note that the sensors used in flow spirometers (e.g. pneumotachographs) are generally held close to the mouth, so expired gas will not have cooled fully before passing from the lung to the sensor. For this and other reasons (e.g. some sensors are heated), the ATPS to BTPS correction equation above may not be appropriate. Under these circumstances, the correct factor should have been determined by the manufacturer and validated and is usually applied automatically; it may also include the effect of temperature and gas composition on the viscosity and density of expired air.

Table B.1 lists the appropriate corrections over the temperature range 17°C to 32°C assuming the expired gas entering the spirometer is fully saturated and that the barometric pressure is 760 mmHg. The correction factors assume that expired gas cools instantly to spirometer temperature. (Note: At sea level, day-to-day variations in barometric pressure do not significantly affect the magnitude of the BTPS correction factor (Johns et al. 2004).)

TABLE B.1	Conversion factors from ATPS to BTPS	
Spirometer temperature (Celsius)	Saturated water vapour (mmHg)	BTPS factor
17	14.5	1.118
18	15.5	1.113
19	16.5	1.108
20	17.5	1.102
21	18.7	1.096
22	19.8	1.091
23	21.1	1.085
24	22.4	1.080
25	23.8	1.075
26	25.2	1.069
27	26.7	1.063
28	28.3	1.057
29	30.0	1.051
30	31.8	1.045
31	33.7	1.039
32	35.7	1.032

Assumes a barometric pressure of 760 mmHg

PREDICTED NORMAL VALUES

The use of a fixed per cent of predicted (e.g. 80%) to define the lower limit of normal (LLN) is widespread despite being shown to be statistically invalid. A more appropriate approach is based on the use of the residual standard deviation (RSD) from regression analyses (usually multiple variables are regressed, that is, age and height), but this is only possible if the survey population data are normally distributed for subjects of all ages and heights. This is because most predicted normal data is homoscedastic, that is, variation in these parameters is uniform across the age and height ranges. The addition or subtraction of 1.64 times the RSD from the mean predicted value results in an upper (or lower, but not both) limit of normality with a confidence level such that 95% of the subjects in the survey lie above the lower limit.

MEAN PREDICTED NORMAL VALUES AND LOWER LIMIT OF NORMAL

Mean predicted and LLN of Caucasian males and females are given in the following tables. The reference data for FEV_1, FVC, FEV_1/FVC and $FEF_{25-75\%}$ cover the age range 4 to 80 years and are based on the work of Stanojevic et al. (2009).[1] The adult reference data for indices based on a 6-second forced expiration (FVC_6, FEV_1/FVC_6 and $FEF_{25-75\%}$) were compiled from data published by Hankinson, Crapo and Jensen (2003). Predicted PEF values for adults and children (aged 8–80 years) were from Hankinson, Odencrantz and Fedan (1999). Age is in years; height in centimetres.

---

1. We are very grateful to Sanja Stanojevic and her colleagues for providing the data for the FEV_1, FVC, FEV_1/FVC and $FEF_{25-75\%}$ predicted normal tables and for permission to include them in our book.

TABLE C.1	Predicted normal values: mean and lower limit of normal — FVC (L) MALE																									
Age (yrs)	20		25		30		35		40		45		50		55		60		65		70		75		80	
	Mean	LLN	Mean	LLN	Mean	LLN	Mean	LLN	Mean	LLN	Mean	LLN	Mean	LLN	Mean	LLN	Mean	LLN	Mean	LLN	Mean	LLN	Mean	LLN	Mean	LLN
145 cm	3.33	2.75	3.39	2.81	3.33	2.75	3.26	2.68	3.20	2.61	3.14	2.54	3.08	2.47	3.00	2.39	2.92	2.29	2.81	2.19	2.69	2.07	2.57	1.95	2.45	1.85
150 cm	3.61	2.99	3.68	3.05	3.62	2.99	3.54	2.91	3.48	2.84	3.41	2.76	3.34	2.68	3.26	2.59	3.17	2.49	3.05	2.37	2.92	2.25	2.79	2.12	2.66	2.01
155 cm	3.91	3.24	3.99	3.30	3.92	3.24	3.84	3.15	3.77	3.07	3.70	2.99	3.62	2.90	3.54	2.81	3.43	2.70	3.31	2.57	3.16	2.43	3.02	2.30	2.89	2.17
160 cm	4.23	3.50	4.31	3.57	4.23	3.50	4.14	3.40	4.07	3.32	3.99	3.23	3.91	3.14	3.82	3.03	3.71	2.92	3.57	2.78	3.42	2.63	3.26	2.48	3.12	2.35
165 cm	4.56	3.77	4.64	3.84	4.56	3.77	4.47	3.67	4.39	3.58	4.31	3.48	4.22	3.38	4.12	3.27	4.00	3.14	3.85	3.00	3.68	2.83	3.51	2.68	3.36	2.53
170 cm	4.90	4.06	4.99	4.13	4.91	4.05	4.80	3.95	4.72	3.85	4.63	3.75	4.53	3.63	4.43	3.51	4.30	3.38	4.14	3.22	3.96	3.05	3.78	2.88	3.61	2.72
175 cm	5.26	4.35	5.36	4.44	5.27	4.35	5.16	4.23	5.06	4.13	4.97	4.02	4.87	3.90	4.75	3.77	4.62	3.63	4.45	3.46	4.25	3.27	4.06	3.09	3.88	2.92
180 cm	5.63	4.66	5.74	4.75	5.64	4.66	5.52	4.53	5.42	4.42	5.32	4.31	5.21	4.18	5.09	4.04	4.94	3.88	4.76	3.70	4.55	3.50	4.34	3.31	4.15	3.13
185 cm	6.02	4.98	6.14	5.08	6.03	4.98	5.90	4.85	5.80	4.73	5.69	4.60	5.57	4.47	5.44	4.32	5.29	4.15	5.09	3.96	4.87	3.75	4.64	3.54	4.44	3.35
190 cm	6.43	5.32	6.55	5.42	6.44	5.31	6.30	5.17	6.18	5.04	6.07	4.91	5.95	4.77	5.81	4.61	5.64	4.43	5.43	4.22	5.19	4.00	4.96	3.77	4.74	3.57
195 cm	6.85	5.67	6.97	5.78	6.86	5.66	6.71	5.51	6.59	5.37	6.47	5.23	6.33	5.08	6.18	4.91	6.01	4.72	5.79	4.50	5.53	4.26	5.28	4.02	5.05	3.80

Source: Stanojevic et al. (2009).

TABLE C.2	Predicted normal values: mean and lower limit of normal FEV₁ (L) MALE																									
Age (yrs)	20		25		30		35		40		45		50		55		60		65		70		75		80	
	Mean	LLN	Mean	LLN	Mean	LLN	Mean	LLN	Mean	LLN	Mean	LLN	Mean	LLN	Mean	LLN	Mean	LLN	Mean	LLN	Mean	LLN	Mean	LLN	Mean	LLN
145 cm	2.83	2.31	2.85	2.33	2.77	2.26	2.68	2.17	2.60	2.09	2.53	2.01	2.44	1.91	2.34	1.81	2.23	1.70	2.12	1.59	2.00	1.47	1.89	1.37	1.78	1.27
150 cm	3.06	2.50	3.08	2.52	3.00	2.44	2.91	2.35	2.82	2.26	2.73	2.17	2.64	2.07	2.53	1.96	2.42	1.84	2.29	1.72	2.16	1.59	2.04	1.48	1.93	1.37
155 cm	3.30	2.70	3.33	2.72	3.24	2.64	3.14	2.54	3.04	2.44	2.95	2.34	2.85	2.24	2.74	2.12	2.61	1.99	2.47	1.85	2.34	1.72	2.21	1.60	2.09	1.48
160 cm	3.56	2.91	3.59	2.93	3.49	2.84	3.38	2.73	3.28	2.63	3.18	2.52	3.07	2.41	2.95	2.28	2.81	2.14	2.67	2.00	2.52	1.85	2.38	1.72	2.25	1.60
165 cm	3.82	3.12	3.86	3.15	3.75	3.05	3.63	2.94	3.52	2.83	3.42	2.71	3.30	2.59	3.17	2.45	3.02	2.30	2.86	2.15	2.70	1.99	2.55	1.85	2.41	1.72
170 cm	4.10	3.35	4.13	3.38	4.02	3.27	3.89	3.15	3.78	3.03	3.66	2.91	3.54	2.77	3.40	2.63	3.24	2.47	3.07	2.30	2.90	2.14	2.74	1.98	2.59	1.84
175 cm	4.39	3.58	4.42	3.61	4.30	3.50	4.17	3.37	4.04	3.25	3.92	3.11	3.79	2.97	3.63	2.81	3.47	2.64	3.29	2.46	3.10	2.29	2.93	2.12	2.77	1.97
180 cm	4.69	3.83	4.73	3.86	4.60	3.74	4.45	3.60	4.32	3.47	4.19	3.33	4.04	3.17	3.88	3.00	3.70	2.82	3.51	2.63	3.31	2.44	3.13	2.26	2.96	2.10
185 cm	5.00	4.08	5.04	4.11	4.90	3.99	4.75	3.84	4.60	3.70	4.46	3.55	4.31	3.38	4.14	3.20	3.95	3.01	3.74	2.81	3.53	2.60	3.34	2.41	3.16	2.24
190 cm	5.32	4.34	5.36	4.38	5.22	4.25	5.05	4.09	4.90	3.93	4.75	3.77	4.59	3.60	4.41	3.41	4.20	3.20	3.98	2.99	3.76	2.77	3.55	2.57	3.36	2.39
195 cm	5.65	4.62	5.70	4.65	5.54	4.51	5.37	4.34	5.21	4.18	5.05	4.01	4.88	3.82	4.68	3.62	4.47	3.40	4.23	3.17	4.00	2.95	3.77	2.73	3.57	2.54

Source: Stanojevic et al. (2009).

TABLE C.3 Predicted normal values: mean and lower limit of normal
FEV₁/FVC MALE

Age (yrs)	20 Mean	20 LLN	25 Mean	25 LLN	30 Mean	30 LLN	35 Mean	35 LLN	40 Mean	40 LLN	45 Mean	45 LLN	50 Mean	50 LLN	55 Mean	55 LLN	60 Mean	60 LLN	65 Mean	65 LLN	70 Mean	70 LLN	75 Mean	75 LLN	80 Mean	80 LLN
145 cm	0.85	0.71	0.83	0.70	0.82	0.69	0.81	0.67	0.80	0.66	0.79	0.65	0.78	0.64	0.78	0.63	0.77	0.62	0.76	0.61	0.76	0.60	0.75	0.59	0.75	0.58
150 cm	0.85	0.71	0.83	0.70	0.82	0.68	0.81	0.67	0.80	0.66	0.79	0.65	0.78	0.64	0.78	0.63	0.77	0.62	0.76	0.61	0.75	0.60	0.75	0.59	0.75	0.58
155 cm	0.85	0.71	0.83	0.70	0.82	0.68	0.81	0.67	0.80	0.66	0.79	0.65	0.78	0.64	0.77	0.63	0.77	0.62	0.76	0.61	0.75	0.60	0.75	0.59	0.75	0.58
160 cm	0.85	0.71	0.83	0.70	0.82	0.68	0.81	0.67	0.80	0.66	0.79	0.65	0.78	0.64	0.77	0.63	0.77	0.62	0.76	0.61	0.75	0.60	0.75	0.59	0.75	0.58
165 cm	0.85	0.71	0.83	0.70	0.82	0.68	0.81	0.67	0.80	0.66	0.79	0.65	0.78	0.64	0.77	0.63	0.77	0.62	0.76	0.61	0.75	0.60	0.75	0.59	0.74	0.58
170 cm	0.85	0.71	0.83	0.70	0.82	0.68	0.81	0.67	0.80	0.66	0.79	0.65	0.78	0.64	0.77	0.63	0.76	0.62	0.76	0.61	0.75	0.60	0.75	0.59	0.74	0.53
175 cm	0.84	0.71	0.83	0.69	0.82	0.68	0.81	0.67	0.80	0.66	0.79	0.65	0.78	0.64	0.77	0.63	0.76	0.62	0.76	0.61	0.75	0.60	0.75	0.59	0.74	0.58
180 cm	0.84	0.71	0.83	0.69	0.82	0.68	0.80	0.67	0.80	0.66	0.79	0.65	0.78	0.64	0.77	0.63	0.76	0.61	0.76	0.60	0.75	0.60	0.75	0.59	0.74	0.58
185 cm	0.84	0.71	0.83	0.69	0.81	0.68	0.80	0.67	0.79	0.66	0.79	0.65	0.78	0.64	0.77	0.63	0.76	0.61	0.76	0.60	0.75	0.59	0.75	0.59	0.74	0.58
190 cm	0.84	0.71	0.83	0.69	0.81	0.68	0.80	0.67	0.79	0.66	0.79	0.65	0.78	0.64	0.77	0.62	0.76	0.61	0.75	0.60	0.75	0.59	0.74	0.59	0.74	0.58
195 cm	0.84	0.71	0.83	0.69	0.81	0.68	0.80	0.67	0.79	0.66	0.79	0.65	0.78	0.64	0.77	0.62	0.76	0.61	0.75	0.60	0.75	0.59	0.74	0.59	0.74	0.58

Source: Stanojevic et al. (2009).

TABLE C.4	Predicted normal values: mean and lower limit of normal FEF$_{25-75\%}$ (L/sec) MALE																									
Age (yrs)	**20**		**25**		**30**		**35**		**40**		**45**		**50**		**55**		**60**		**65**		**70**		**75**		**80**	
	Mean	LLN	Mean	LLN	Mean	LLN	Mean	LLN	Mean	LLN	Mean	LLN	Mean	LLN	Mean	LLN	Mean	LLN	Mean	LLN	Mean	LLN	Mean	LLN	Mean	LLN
145 cm	3.24	2.12	3.19	2.09	3.04	1.97	2.91	1.85	2.80	1.73	2.65	1.60	2.46	1.42	2.23	1.24	1.99	1.05	1.74	0.87	1.52	0.71	1.36	0.58	1.24	0.49
150 cm	3.45	2.26	3.40	2.22	3.24	2.09	3.09	1.97	2.97	1.84	2.82	1.70	2.61	1.51	2.37	1.31	2.11	1.11	1.85	0.92	1.62	0.75	1.44	0.62	1.32	0.52
155 cm	3.66	2.39	3.60	2.35	3.43	2.22	3.28	2.09	3.15	1.96	2.99	1.80	2.77	1.61	2.51	1.39	2.24	1.18	1.97	0.98	1.72	0.80	1.53	0.66	1.40	0.55
160 cm	3.87	2.53	3.82	2.49	3.64	2.35	3.47	2.21	3.34	2.07	3.17	1.91	2.93	1.70	2.66	1.48	2.37	1.25	2.08	1.04	1.82	0.85	1.62	0.70	1.48	0.58
165 cm	4.10	2.68	4.03	2.63	3.84	2.49	3.67	2.33	3.53	2.19	3.35	2.01	3.10	1.80	2.81	1.56	2.51	1.32	2.20	1.10	1.92	0.90	1.71	0.74	1.57	0.61
170 cm	4.32	2.83	4.26	2.78	4.06	2.63	3.87	2.46	3.73	2.31	3.54	2.13	3.27	1.90	2.97	1.65	2.65	1.40	2.33	1.16	2.03	1.00	1.81	0.78	1.65	0.65
175 cm	4.56	2.98	4.49	2.93	4.28	2.77	4.08	2.60	3.93	2.44	3.73	2.24	3.45	2.00	3.13	1.74	2.79	1.47	2.45	1.22	2.14	1.00	1.91	0.82	1.74	0.68
180 cm	4.79	3.14	4.72	3.08	4.50	2.91	4.30	2.73	4.13	2.56	3.92	2.36	3.63	2.10	3.29	1.83	2.94	1.55	2.58	1.28	2.25	1.05	2.01	0.86	1.83	0.72
185 cm	5.04	3.29	4.96	3.24	4.73	3.06	4.51	2.87	4.34	2.69	4.12	2.48	3.82	2.21	3.46	1.92	3.08	1.63	2.71	1.35	2.37	1.10	2.11	0.91	1.93	0.76
190 cm	5.28	3.46	5.21	3.40	4.96	3.21	4.74	3.01	4.56	2.83	4.33	2.60	4.00	2.32	3.63	2.01	3.24	1.71	2.84	1.42	2.48	1.16	2.21	0.95	2.02	0.79
195 cm	5.54	3.62	5.46	3.56	5.20	3.36	4.96	3.16	4.77	2.96	4.53	2.72	4.20	2.43	3.80	2.11	3.39	1.79	2.98	1.48	2.60	1.21	2.32	1.00	2.12	0.83

Source: Stanojevic et al. (2009).

TABLE C.5	Predicated normal values: mean and lower limit of normal PEF (L/min) MALE																										
Age (yrs)	20		25		30		35		40		45		50		55		60		65		70		75		80	
	Mean	LLN	Mean	LLN	Mean	LLN	Mean	LLN	Mean	LLN	Mean	LLN	Mean	LLN	Mean	LLN	Mean	LLN	Mean	LLN	Mean	LLN	Mean	LLN	Mean	LLN
145 cm	446	354	453	361	457	364	456	364	452	359	443	351	431	339	415	322	395	302	371	278	343	251	311	219	276	193
150 cm	468	369	475	377	479	380	478	379	474	375	465	366	453	354	437	338	417	318	393	294	365	266	333	234	298	209
155 cm	491	385	498	393	502	396	501	395	497	391	488	383	476	370	460	354	440	334	416	310	388	282	356	250	320	215
160 cm	515	402	522	409	525	413	525	412	520	408	512	399	500	387	483	371	463	351	439	327	411	299	380	267	344	231
165 cm	539	419	546	426	550	430	549	429	545	425	536	416	524	404	508	388	488	368	464	344	436	316	404	284	368	249
170 cm	564	437	571	444	575	448	574	447	570	443	561	434	549	422	533	406	513	386	489	362	461	334	429	302	393	266
175 cm	590	455	597	462	600	466	600	465	595	461	587	452	575	440	559	424	539	404	515	380	487	352	455	320	419	285
180 cm	616	474	624	481	627	485	626	484	622	480	614	471	601	459	585	443	565	423	541	399	513	371	482	339	446	303
185 cm	644	493	651	501	654	504	654	503	649	499	641	491	629	478	613	462	593	442	569	418	541	390	509	358	473	323
190 cm	672	513	679	520	682	524	682	523	677	519	669	510	657	498	641	482	621	462	597	438	569	410	537	378	501	343
195 cm	701	534	708	541	711	544	711	544	706	539	698	531	686	518	669	502	649	482	625	458	598	430	566	399	530	363

Source: Hankinson, Odencrantz & Fedan (1999).

| TABLE C.6 | Predicated normal values: mean and lower limit of normal FVC₆ (L) MALE |

Age (yrs)	20 Mean	20 LLN	25 Mean	25 LLN	30 Mean	30 LLN	35 Mean	35 LLN	40 Mean	40 LLN	45 Mean	45 LLN	50 Mean	50 LLN	55 Mean	55 LLN	60 Mean	60 LLN	65 Mean	65 LLN	70 Mean	70 LLN	75 Mean	75 LLN	80 Mean	80 LLN
145 cm	3.67	3.06	3.58	2.97	3.48	2.87	3.37	2.76	3.24	2.64	3.10	2.50	2.96	2.35	2.80	2.19	2.63	2.02	2.44	1.84	2.25	1.64	2.04	1.44	1.82	1.22
150 cm	3.94	3.29	3.85	3.20	3.75	3.10	3.63	2.99	3.51	2.86	3.37	2.72	3.23	2.58	3.07	2.42	2.89	2.25	2.71	2.06	2.52	1.87	2.31	1.66	2.09	1.44
155 cm	4.21	3.52	4.12	3.43	4.02	3.33	3.91	3.22	3.79	3.09	3.65	2.96	3.50	2.81	3.34	2.65	3.17	2.48	2.99	2.30	2.79	2.10	2.59	1.90	2.37	1.68
160 cm	4.50	3.76	4.41	3.67	4.31	3.57	4.20	3.46	4.07	3.33	3.94	3.20	3.79	3.05	3.63	2.89	3.46	2.72	3.27	2.54	3.08	2.34	2.87	2.14	2.66	1.92
165 cm	4.80	4.01	4.71	3.92	4.60	3.82	4.49	3.71	4.37	3.58	4.23	3.45	4.08	3.30	3.92	3.14	3.75	2.97	3.57	2.79	3.38	2.59	3.17	2.38	2.95	2.17
170 cm	5.10	4.27	5.01	4.18	4.91	4.08	4.80	3.96	4.67	3.84	4.54	3.70	4.39	3.56	4.23	3.40	4.06	3.22	3.87	3.04	3.68	2.85	3.47	2.64	3.26	2.42
175 cm	5.41	4.53	5.32	4.44	5.22	4.34	5.11	4.23	4.99	4.10	4.85	3.97	4.70	3.82	4.54	3.66	4.37	3.49	4.19	3.31	3.99	3.11	3.79	2.90	3.57	2.69
180 cm	5.74	4.80	5.65	4.71	5.55	4.61	5.43	4.50	5.31	4.37	5.17	4.24	5.02	4.09	4.86	3.93	4.69	3.76	4.51	3.58	4.32	3.38	4.11	3.18	3.89	2.96
185 cm	6.07	5.08	5.98	4.99	5.88	4.89	5.76	4.78	5.64	4.65	5.50	4.52	5.36	4.37	5.20	4.21	5.02	4.04	4.84	3.86	4.65	3.66	4.44	3.45	4.22	3.24
190 cm	6.41	5.37	6.32	5.28	6.22	5.18	6.10	5.06	5.98	4.94	5.84	4.80	5.70	4.66	5.54	4.50	5.37	4.33	5.18	4.14	4.99	3.95	4.78	3.74	4.56	3.52
195 cm	6.76	5.66	6.67	5.57	6.57	5.47	6.45	5.36	6.33	5.23	6.19	5.10	6.05	4.95	5.89	4.79	5.72	4.62	5.53	4.44	5.34	4.24	5.13	4.04	4.91	3.82

Source: Hankinson, Crapo & Jensen (2003).

TABLE C.7	Predicated normal values: mean and lower limit of normal FEV$_1$/FVC$_6$ MALE																				
Age (yrs)	20		25		30		35		40		45		50		55		60		65		70		75		80	
	Mean	LLN	Mean	LLN	Mean	LLN	Mean	LLN	Mean	LLN	Mean	LLN	Mean	LLN	Mean	LLN	Mean	LLN	Mean	LLN	Mean	LLN	Mean	LLN	Mean	LLN
All heights	0.85	0.76	0.84	0.75	0.82	0.74	0.82	0.73	0.82	0.72	0.81	0.72	0.80	0.71	0.80	0.71	0.79	0.70	0.78	0.69	0.78	0.69	0.77	0.68	0.76	0.67

Source: Hankinson, Crapo & Jensen (2003).

TABLE C.8	Predicated normal values: mean and lower limit of normal FEF$_{25-75\%}$ (L/sec) MALE																									
Age (yrs)	20		25		30		35		40		45		50		55		60		65		70		75		80	
	Mean	LLN	Mean	LLN	Mean	LLN	Mean	LLN	Mean	LLN	Mean	LLN	Mean	LLN	Mean	LLN	Mean	LLN	Mean	LLN	Mean	LLN	Mean	LLN	Mean	LLN
145 cm	3.81	2.69	3.61	2.49	3.41	2.29	3.21	2.09	3.01	1.89	2.81	1.69	2.61	1.49	2.41	1.29	2.21	1.09	2.01	0.89	1.81	0.69	1.61	0.49	1.41	0.29
150 cm	3.98	2.78	3.78	2.58	3.58	2.38	3.38	2.18	3.18	1.98	2.98	1.78	2.78	1.58	2.58	1.38	2.38	1.18	2.18	0.98	1.98	0.78	1.78	0.58	1.58	0.38
155 cm	4.15	2.88	3.95	2.68	3.75	2.48	3.55	2.28	3.35	2.08	3.15	1.88	2.95	1.68	2.75	1.48	2.55	1.28	2.35	1.08	2.15	0.88	1.95	0.68	1.75	0.48
160 cm	4.33	2.97	4.13	2.77	3.93	2.57	3.73	2.37	3.53	2.17	3.33	1.97	3.13	1.77	2.93	1.57	2.73	1.37	2.53	1.17	2.33	0.97	2.13	0.77	1.93	0.57
165 cm	4.52	3.07	4.32	2.87	4.12	2.67	3.92	2.47	3.72	2.27	3.52	2.07	3.32	1.87	3.12	1.67	2.92	1.47	2.72	1.27	2.52	1.07	2.32	0.87	2.12	0.67
170 cm	4.71	3.18	4.51	2.98	4.31	2.78	4.11	2.58	3.91	2.38	3.71	2.18	3.51	1.98	3.31	1.78	3.11	1.58	2.91	1.38	2.71	1.18	2.51	0.98	2.31	0.78
175 cm	4.91	3.28	4.71	3.08	4.51	2.88	4.31	2.68	4.11	2.48	3.91	2.28	3.71	2.08	3.51	1.88	3.31	1.68	3.11	1.48	2.91	1.28	2.71	1.08	2.51	0.88
180 cm	5.11	3.39	4.91	3.19	4.71	2.99	4.51	2.79	4.31	2.59	4.11	2.39	3.91	2.19	3.71	1.99	3.51	1.79	3.31	1.59	3.11	1.39	2.91	1.19	2.71	0.99
185 cm	5.32	3.51	5.12	3.31	4.92	3.11	4.72	2.91	4.52	2.71	4.32	2.51	4.12	2.31	3.92	2.11	3.72	1.91	3.52	1.71	3.32	1.51	3.12	1.31	2.92	1.11
190 cm	5.54	3.62	5.34	3.42	5.14	3.22	4.94	3.02	4.74	2.82	4.54	2.62	4.34	2.42	4.14	2.22	3.94	2.02	3.74	1.82	3.54	1.62	3.34	1.42	3.14	1.22
195 cm	5.76	3.74	5.56	3.54	5.36	3.34	5.16	3.14	4.96	2.94	4.76	2.74	4.56	2.54	4.36	2.34	4.16	2.14	3.96	1.94	3.76	1.74	3.56	1.54	3.36	1.34

Source: Hankinson, Crapo & Jensen (2003).

TABLE C.9 Predicted normal values: mean and lower limit of normal
FVC (L) FEMALE

Age (yrs)	20 Mean	20 LLN	25 Mean	25 LLN	30 Mean	30 LLN	35 Mean	35 LLN	40 Mean	40 LLN	45 Mean	45 LLN	50 Mean	50 LLN	55 Mean	55 LLN	60 Mean	60 LLN	65 Mean	65 LLN	70 Mean	70 LLN	75 Mean	75 LLN	80 Mean	80 LLN
145 cm	2.87	2.37	2.92	2.41	2.92	2.40	2.89	2.38	2.85	2.33	2.78	2.25	2.68	2.15	2.58	2.03	2.47	1.91	2.36	1.79	2.25	1.67	2.15	1.56	2.06	1.46
150 cm	3.11	2.56	3.16	2.61	3.16	2.60	3.13	2.57	3.08	2.52	3.01	2.43	2.90	2.32	2.79	2.20	2.67	2.07	2.55	1.94	2.44	1.81	2.33	1.69	2.23	1.58
155 cm	3.35	2.77	3.41	2.81	3.41	2.81	3.38	2.78	3.33	2.72	3.24	2.63	3.13	2.51	3.01	2.37	2.88	2.23	2.76	2.09	2.63	1.95	2.51	1.82	2.41	1.70
160 cm	3.61	2.98	3.67	3.03	3.67	3.02	3.64	2.99	3.59	2.93	3.49	2.83	3.37	2.70	3.24	2.55	3.10	2.40	2.97	2.25	2.83	2.10	2.71	1.96	2.59	1.83
165 cm	3.88	3.20	3.94	3.25	3.94	3.25	3.91	3.22	3.85	3.15	3.75	3.04	3.63	2.90	3.48	2.74	3.33	2.58	3.19	2.42	3.05	2.26	2.91	2.11	2.78	1.97
170 cm	4.16	3.43	4.23	3.49	4.23	3.48	4.20	3.45	4.13	3.38	4.03	3.26	3.89	3.11	3.73	2.94	3.58	2.77	3.42	2.59	3.27	2.42	3.12	2.26	2.98	2.11
175 cm	4.45	3.67	4.52	3.73	4.52	3.73	4.49	3.69	4.42	3.61	4.31	3.49	4.16	3.33	4.00	3.15	3.83	2.96	3.66	2.77	3.49	2.59	3.34	2.42	3.19	2.26
180 cm	4.75	3.92	4.83	3.99	4.83	3.98	4.79	3.94	4.72	3.86	4.60	3.73	4.44	3.55	4.27	3.36	4.09	3.16	3.91	2.96	3.73	2.77	3.57	2.59	3.41	2.42
185 cm	5.07	4.18	5.15	4.25	5.15	4.24	5.11	4.20	5.03	4.11	4.90	3.97	4.74	3.79	4.55	3.58	4.36	3.37	4.16	3.16	3.98	2.95	3.80	2.76	3.63	2.57
190 cm	5.39	4.45	5.48	4.52	5.48	4.52	5.44	4.47	5.36	4.38	5.22	4.23	5.04	4.03	4.84	3.81	4.64	3.59	4.43	3.36	4.23	3.14	4.04	2.93	3.87	2.74
195 cm	5.73	4.73	5.82	4.81	5.82	4.80	5.78	4.75	5.69	4.65	5.54	4.49	5.35	4.28	5.14	4.05	4.92	3.81	4.71	3.57	4.50	3.34	4.30	3.12	4.11	2.91

Source: Stanojevic et al. (2009).

TABLE C.10	Predicted normal values: mean and lower limit of normal FEV$_1$ (L) FEMALE																									
Age (yrs)	20		25		30		35		40		45		50		55		60		65		70		75		80	
	Mean	LLN	Mean	LLN	Mean	LLN	Mean	LLN	Mean	LLN	Mean	LLN	Mean	LLN	Mean	LLN	Mean	LLN	Mean	LLN	Mean	LLN	Mean	LLN	Mean	LLN
145 cm	2.54	2.06	2.54	2.06	2.50	2.02	2.44	1.96	2.36	1.89	2.27	1.80	2.16	1.71	2.05	1.60	1.94	1.50	1.83	1.41	1.73	1.32	1.64	1.24	1.55	1.16
150 cm	2.74	2.22	2.74	2.22	2.69	2.18	2.63	2.11	2.55	2.04	2.45	1.94	2.33	1.84	2.21	1.73	2.09	1.62	1.97	1.51	1.86	1.42	1.76	1.33	1.67	1.25
155 cm	2.95	2.39	2.95	2.39	2.89	2.34	2.82	2.27	2.74	2.19	2.63	2.09	2.50	1.98	2.37	1.86	2.24	1.74	2.12	1.63	2.00	1.53	1.89	1.43	1.80	1.35
160 cm	3.16	2.56	3.16	2.56	3.10	2.51	3.03	2.44	2.93	2.35	2.82	2.24	2.69	2.12	2.55	1.99	2.40	1.86	2.27	1.75	2.15	1.64	2.03	1.54	1.93	1.44
165 cm	3.38	2.74	3.38	2.74	3.32	2.68	3.24	2.61	3.14	2.51	3.02	2.40	2.87	2.27	2.72	2.13	2.57	2.00	2.43	1.87	2.30	1.75	2.17	1.64	2.06	1.54
170 cm	3.61	2.92	3.61	2.92	3.54	2.87	3.46	2.78	3.35	2.68	3.22	2.56	3.07	2.42	2.91	2.28	2.75	2.13	2.59	1.99	2.45	1.87	2.32	1.75	2.20	1.65
175 cm	3.85	3.12	3.85	3.12	3.78	3.05	3.69	2.97	3.57	2.86	3.43	2.73	3.27	2.58	3.10	2.42	2.93	2.27	2.77	2.13	2.61	1.99	2.47	1.87	2.35	1.76
180 cm	4.09	3.32	4.09	3.32	4.02	3.25	3.92	3.16	3.80	3.04	3.65	2.90	3.48	2.74	3.30	2.58	3.11	2.42	2.94	2.26	2.78	2.12	2.63	1.99	2.50	1.87
185 cm	4.35	3.52	4.35	3.52	4.27	3.45	4.16	3.35	4.04	3.23	3.88	3.08	3.70	2.92	3.50	2.74	3.31	2.57	3.12	2.40	2.95	2.25	2.80	2.11	2.65	1.99
190 cm	4.61	3.73	4.61	3.73	4.53	3.66	4.42	3.56	4.28	3.43	4.11	3.27	3.92	3.09	3.71	2.91	3.51	2.72	3.31	2.55	3.13	2.39	2.96	2.24	2.81	2.11
195 cm	4.88	3.95	4.88	3.95	4.79	3.87	4.68	3.76	4.53	3.63	4.35	3.46	4.15	3.27	3.93	3.08	3.71	2.88	3.51	2.70	3.32	2.53	3.14	2.37	2.98	2.23

Source: Stanojevic et al. (2009).

TABLE C.11 Predicted normal values: mean and lower limit of normal
FEV₁/FVC FEMALE

Age (yrs)	20 Mean	20 LLN	25 Mean	25 LLN	30 Mean	30 LLN	35 Mean	35 LLN	40 Mean	40 LLN	45 Mean	45 LLN	50 Mean	50 LLN	55 Mean	55 LLN	60 Mean	60 LLN	65 Mean	65 LLN	70 Mean	70 LLN	75 Mean	75 LLN	80 Mean	80 LLN
145 cm	0.89	0.77	0.88	0.76	0.86	0.74	0.84	0.73	0.83	0.71	0.82	0.70	0.80	0.68	0.79	0.66	0.79	0.65	0.78	0.63	0.78	0.62	0.78	0.61	0.77	0.59
150 cm	0.89	0.77	0.87	0.75	0.86	0.74	0.84	0.72	0.83	0.71	0.81	0.69	0.80	0.68	0.79	0.66	0.78	0.65	0.78	0.63	0.77	0.62	0.77	0.61	0.77	0.59
155 cm	0.89	0.77	0.87	0.75	0.86	0.74	0.84	0.72	0.83	0.71	0.81	0.69	0.80	0.68	0.79	0.66	0.78	0.64	0.78	0.63	0.77	0.62	0.77	0.60	0.77	0.59
160 cm	0.88	0.76	0.87	0.75	0.85	0.74	0.84	0.72	0.82	0.71	0.81	0.69	0.80	0.67	0.79	0.66	0.78	0.64	0.77	0.63	0.77	0.62	0.77	0.60	0.77	0.59
165 cm	0.88	0.76	0.87	0.75	0.85	0.73	0.84	0.72	0.82	0.70	0.81	0.69	0.80	0.67	0.79	0.66	0.78	0.64	0.77	0.63	0.77	0.61	0.77	0.60	0.77	0.59
170 cm	0.88	0.76	0.87	0.75	0.85	0.73	0.83	0.72	0.82	0.70	0.81	0.69	0.79	0.67	0.78	0.66	0.78	0.64	0.77	0.63	0.77	0.61	0.77	0.60	0.76	0.59
175 cm	0.88	0.76	0.86	0.75	0.85	0.73	0.83	0.72	0.82	0.70	0.80	0.68	0.79	0.67	0.78	0.65	0.77	0.64	0.77	0.62	0.77	0.61	0.76	0.60	0.76	0.59
180 cm	0.88	0.76	0.86	0.74	0.85	0.73	0.83	0.71	0.82	0.70	0.80	0.68	0.79	0.67	0.78	0.65	0.77	0.64	0.77	0.62	0.76	0.61	0.76	0.60	0.76	0.53
185 cm	0.87	0.75	0.86	0.74	0.84	0.73	0.83	0.71	0.81	0.70	0.80	0.68	0.79	0.67	0.78	0.65	0.77	0.64	0.76	0.62	0.76	0.61	0.76	0.60	0.76	0.53
190 cm	0.87	0.75	0.86	0.74	0.84	0.73	0.83	0.71	0.81	0.70	0.80	0.68	0.79	0.66	0.78	0.65	0.77	0.63	0.76	0.62	0.76	0.61	0.76	0.60	0.76	0.53
195 cm	0.87	0.75	0.86	0.74	0.84	0.72	0.83	0.71	0.81	0.69	0.80	0.68	0.78	0.66	0.77	0.65	0.77	0.63	0.76	0.62	0.76	0.61	0.75	0.59	0.76	0.58

Source: Stanojevic et al. (2009).

TABLE C.12	Predicted normal values: mean and lower limit of normal FEF 25-75% (L/sec) FEMALE																									
Age (yrs)	20		25		30		35		40		45		50		55		60		65		70		75		80	
	Mean	LLN	Mean	LLN	Mean	LLN	Mean	LLN	Mean	LLN	Mean	LLN	Mean	LLN	Mean	LLN	Mean	LLN	Mean	LLN	Mean	LLN	Mean	LLN	Mean	LLN
145 cm	3.13	2.06	3.07	2.00	2.92	1.88	2.75	1.74	2.57	1.58	2.38	1.41	2.18	1.24	1.99	1.08	1.81	0.94	1.65	0.81	1.51	0.70	1.39	0.60	1.29	0.52
150 cm	3.30	2.18	3.24	2.11	3.09	1.99	2.91	1.84	2.71	1.67	2.51	1.49	2.30	1.31	2.10	1.14	1.91	0.99	1.74	0.85	1.60	0.74	1.47	0.64	1.36	0.55
155 cm	3.48	2.30	3.42	2.23	3.26	2.10	3.07	1.93	2.86	1.76	2.65	1.57	2.43	1.38	2.21	1.20	2.02	1.04	1.84	0.90	1.69	0.78	1.55	0.67	1.44	0.58
160 cm	3.67	2.42	3.59	2.35	3.43	2.21	3.23	2.04	3.01	1.85	2.79	1.65	2.55	1.46	2.33	1.27	2.12	1.10	1.94	0.95	1.77	0.82	1.63	0.71	1.51	0.61
165 cm	3.85	2.54	3.78	2.47	3.60	2.32	3.39	2.14	3.17	1.94	2.93	1.74	2.68	1.53	2.45	1.33	2.23	1.15	2.03	0.99	1.86	0.86	1.72	0.74	1.59	0.64
170 cm	4.04	2.66	3.96	2.59	3.78	2.43	3.56	2.25	3.32	2.04	3.07	1.82	2.82	1.61	2.57	1.40	2.34	1.21	2.13	1.04	1.96	0.90	1.80	0.78	1.67	0.67
175 cm	4.24	2.79	4.15	2.71	3.96	2.55	3.73	2.35	3.48	2.14	3.22	1.91	2.95	1.68	2.69	1.47	2.45	1.27	2.24	1.09	2.05	0.95	1.89	0.82	1.75	0.71
180 cm	4.43	2.92	4.35	2.84	4.15	2.67	3.90	2.46	3.64	2.24	3.37	2.00	3.09	1.76	2.82	1.53	2.57	1.33	2.34	1.14	2.15	0.99	1.98	0.86	1.83	0.74
185 cm	4.64	3.05	4.54	2.97	4.33	2.79	4.08	2.57	3.81	2.34	3.52	2.09	3.23	1.84	2.95	1.60	2.68	1.39	2.45	1.20	2.24	1.03	2.07	0.89	1.91	0.77
190 cm	4.84	3.16	4.74	3.10	4.52	2.91	4.26	2.69	3.98	2.44	3.68	2.18	3.37	1.92	3.08	1.67	2.80	1.45	2.55	1.25	2.34	1.08	2.16	0.93	1.99	0.81
195 cm	5.05	3.32	4.95	3.23	4.72	3.04	4.44	2.80	4.15	2.55	3.83	2.27	3.52	2.00	3.21	1.74	2.92	1.51	2.66	1.30	2.44	1.13	2.25	0.97	2.08	0.84

Source: Stanojevic et al. (2009).

TABLE C.13	Predicted normal values: mean and lower limit of normal PEF (L/min) FEMALE																												
Age (yrs)	18		20		25		30		35		40		45		50		55		60		65		70		75		80	
	Mean	LLN	Mean	LLN	Mean	LLN	Mean	LLN	Mean	LLN	Mean	LLN	Mean	LLN	Mean	LLN	Mean	LLN	Mean	LLN	Mean	LLN	Mean	LLN	Mean	LLN	Mean	LLN
145 cm	345	264	349	267	356	274	360	278	360	279	358	276	352	271	344	262	332	250	317	236	299	218	278	197	254	173	227	146
150 cm	362	274	365	278	372	285	376	289	377	289	374	287	369	281	360	273	349	261	334	246	316	228	295	208	271	183	244	156
155 cm	379	286	382	289	389	296	393	300	394	300	391	298	386	293	377	284	366	272	351	257	333	240	312	219	288	195	261	167
160 cm	396	297	400	301	407	307	411	311	411	312	409	310	403	304	395	295	383	284	368	269	351	251	330	230	305	206	278	179
165 cm	415	309	418	312	425	319	429	323	430	324	427	321	422	316	413	307	401	296	387	281	369	263	348	242	324	218	296	191
170 cm	433	321	437	325	444	332	448	335	448	336	446	334	440	328	432	319	420	308	405	293	387	275	366	254	342	230	315	203
175 cm	453	334	456	337	463	344	467	348	468	349	465	346	460	341	451	332	439	320	425	306	407	288	386	267	362	243	334	216
180 cm	472	347	476	350	483	357	487	361	487	361	485	359	479	354	471	345	459	333	444	319	427	301	406	280	381	256	354	228
185 cm	493	360	496	363	503	370	507	374	508	375	505	372	500	367	491	358	480	347	465	332	447	314	426	293	402	269	375	242
190 cm	514	374	517	377	524	384	528	388	529	388	526	386	521	381	512	372	501	360	486	345	468	328	447	307	423	283	396	255
195 cm	535	388	539	391	546	398	550	402	550	402	548	400	542	395	534	386	522	374	507	360	489	342	468	321	444	297	417	263

Source: Hankinson, Odencrantz & Fedan (1999).

TABLE C.14	Predicted normal values: mean and lower limit of normal FVC$_6$ (L) FEMALE																											
Age (yrs)	18		20		25		30		35		40		45		50		55		60		65		70		75		80	
	Mean	LLN	Mean	LLN	Mean	LLN	Mean	LLN	Mean	LLN	Mean	LLN	Mean	LLN	Mean	LLN	Mean	LLN	Mean	LLN	Mean	LLN	Mean	LLN	Mean	LLN	Mean	LLN
145 cm	3.00	2.48	3.00	2.47	2.98	2.46	2.95	2.42	2.89	2.37	2.82	2.30	2.74	2.21	2.63	2.11	2.51	1.99	2.37	1.85	2.22	1.70	2.05	1.52	1.86	1.33	1.65	1.13
150 cm	3.22	2.66	3.21	2.65	3.20	2.64	3.16	2.60	3.11	2.55	3.04	2.48	2.95	2.39	2.85	2.29	2.73	2.17	2.59	2.03	2.44	1.88	2.26	1.70	2.07	1.51	1.86	1.30
155 cm	3.44	2.84	3.44	2.84	3.42	2.82	3.39	2.79	3.33	2.74	3.26	2.67	3.18	2.58	3.07	2.48	2.95	2.35	2.81	2.22	2.66	2.06	2.49	1.89	2.30	1.70	2.09	1.49
160 cm	3.67	3.03	3.67	3.03	3.65	3.01	3.62	2.98	3.56	2.93	3.49	2.86	3.41	2.77	3.30	2.67	3.18	2.55	3.04	2.41	2.89	2.25	2.72	2.08	2.53	1.89	2.32	1.68
165 cm	3.91	3.23	3.91	3.23	3.89	3.21	3.85	3.18	3.80	3.12	3.73	3.05	3.65	2.97	3.54	2.86	3.42	2.74	3.28	2.61	3.13	2.45	2.95	2.28	2.76	2.09	2.56	1.88
170 cm	4.15	3.43	4.15	3.43	4.13	3.41	4.10	3.38	4.05	3.33	3.98	3.26	3.89	3.17	3.79	3.07	3.67	2.95	3.53	2.81	3.37	2.65	3.20	2.48	3.01	2.29	2.80	2.08
175 cm	4.41	3.64	4.40	3.64	4.39	3.62	4.35	3.59	4.30	3.54	4.23	3.47	4.14	3.38	4.04	3.28	3.92	3.16	3.78	3.02	3.63	2.86	3.45	2.69	3.26	2.50	3.06	2.29
180 cm	4.67	3.86	4.66	3.86	4.65	3.84	4.61	3.81	4.56	3.75	4.49	3.68	4.40	3.60	4.30	3.49	4.18	3.37	4.04	3.23	3.89	3.08	3.71	2.91	3.52	2.72	3.32	2.51
185 cm	4.93	4.08	4.93	4.08	4.91	4.06	4.88	4.03	4.83	3.98	4.76	3.91	4.67	3.82	4.57	3.72	4.45	3.59	4.31	3.46	4.15	3.30	3.98	3.13	3.79	2.94	3.58	2.73
190 cm	5.21	4.31	5.21	4.31	5.19	4.29	5.15	4.26	5.10	4.20	5.03	4.13	4.95	4.05	4.84	3.94	4.72	3.82	4.58	3.68	4.43	3.53	4.25	3.36	4.06	3.17	3.86	2.96
195 cm	5.49	4.54	5.49	4.54	5.47	4.52	5.44	4.49	5.38	4.44	5.31	4.37	5.23	4.28	5.12	4.18	5.00	4.06	4.87	3.92	4.71	3.76	4.54	3.59	4.35	3.40	4.14	3.19

Source: Hankinson, Crapo & Jensen (2003).

| TABLE C.15 | Predicted normal values: mean and lower limit of normal FEV₁/FVC₆ FEMALE | | | | | | | | | | | | | |

Age (yrs)	18		20		25		30		35		40		45		50		55		60		65		70		75		80	
	Mean	LLN	Mean	LLN	Mean	LLN	Mean	LLN	Mean	LLN	Mean	LLN	Mean	LLN	Mean	LLN	Mean	LLN	Mean	LLN	Mean	LLN	Mean	LLN	Mean	LLN
All heights	0.87	0.79	0.87	0.78	0.86	0.77	0.85	0.77	0.85	0.76	0.84	0.75	0.83	0.74	0.82	0.74	0.81	0.73	0.81	0.72	0.80	0.71	0.79	0.70	0.78	0.70	0.77	0.39

Source: Hankinson, Crapo & Jensen (2003).

TABLE C.16	Predicted normal values: mean and lower limit of normal FEF$_{25-75\%}$ (L/sec) FEMALE																										
Age (yrs)	18		20		25		30		35		40		45		50		55		60		65		70		75		80	
	Mean	LLN	Mean	LLN	Mean	LLN	Mean	LLN	Mean	LLN	Mean	LLN	Mean	LLN	Mean	LLN	Mean	LLN	Mean	LLN	Mean	LLN	Mean	LLN	Mean	LLN	Mean	LLN
145 cm	3.52	2.50	3.45	2.44	3.28	2.27	3.11	2.10	2.94	1.93	2.77	1.76	2.60	1.59	2.43	1.42	2.26	1.25	2.09	1.08	1.92	0.91	1.75	0.74	1.58	0.57	1.41	0.40
150 cm	3.65	2.56	3.58	2.49	3.41	2.32	3.24	2.15	3.07	1.98	2.90	1.81	2.73	1.64	2.56	1.47	2.39	1.30	2.22	1.13	2.05	0.96	1.88	0.79	1.71	0.62	1.54	0.45
155 cm	3.78	2.62	3.71	2.55	3.54	2.38	3.37	2.21	3.20	2.04	3.03	1.87	2.86	1.70	2.69	1.53	2.52	1.36	2.35	1.19	2.18	1.02	2.01	0.85	1.84	0.68	1.67	0.51
160 cm	3.92	2.68	3.85	2.61	3.68	2.44	3.51	2.27	3.34	2.10	3.17	1.93	3.00	1.76	2.83	1.59	2.66	1.42	2.49	1.25	2.32	1.08	2.15	0.91	1.98	0.74	1.81	0.57
165 cm	4.06	2.75	3.99	2.68	3.82	2.51	3.65	2.34	3.48	2.17	3.31	2.00	3.14	1.83	2.97	1.66	2.80	1.49	2.63	1.32	2.46	1.15	2.29	0.98	2.12	0.81	1.95	0.64
170 cm	4.21	2.81	4.14	2.74	3.97	2.57	3.80	2.40	3.63	2.23	3.46	2.06	3.29	1.89	3.12	1.72	2.95	1.55	2.78	1.38	2.61	1.21	2.44	1.04	2.27	0.87	2.10	0.70
175 cm	4.36	2.88	4.29	2.81	4.12	2.64	3.95	2.47	3.78	2.30	3.61	2.13	3.44	1.96	3.27	1.79	3.10	1.62	2.93	1.45	2.76	1.28	2.59	1.11	2.42	0.94	2.25	0.77
180 cm	4.51	2.95	4.44	2.88	4.27	2.71	4.10	2.54	3.93	2.37	3.76	2.20	3.59	2.03	3.42	1.86	3.25	1.69	3.08	1.52	2.91	1.35	2.74	1.18	2.57	1.01	2.40	0.84
185 cm	4.67	3.02	4.60	2.95	4.43	2.78	4.26	2.61	4.09	2.44	3.92	2.27	3.75	2.10	3.58	1.93	3.41	1.76	3.24	1.59	3.07	1.42	2.90	1.25	2.73	1.08	2.56	0.91
190 cm	4.84	3.09	4.77	3.03	4.60	2.86	4.43	2.69	4.26	2.52	4.09	2.35	3.92	2.18	3.75	2.01	3.58	1.84	3.41	1.67	3.24	1.50	3.07	1.33	2.90	1.16	2.73	0.99
195 cm	5.00	3.17	4.94	3.10	4.77	2.93	4.60	2.76	4.43	2.59	4.26	2.42	4.09	2.25	3.92	2.08	3.75	1.91	3.58	1.74	3.41	1.57	3.24	1.40	3.07	1.23	2.90	1.06

Source: Hankinson, Crapo & Jensen (2003).

TABLE C.17	Predicted normal values: mean and lower limit of normal FEV₁ (L) MALE CHILDREN														
Age (yrs)	**4**		**6**		**8**		**10**		**12**		**14**		**16**		**18**	
	Mean	LLN	Mean	LLN	Mean	LLN	Mean	LLN	Mean	LLN	Mean	LLN	Mean	LLN	Mean	LLN
110 cm	1.06	0.79	1.13	0.87	1.14	0.91	–	–	–	–	–	–	–	–	–	–
115 cm	1.18	0.88	1.25	0.97	1.27	1.01	1.27	1.02	–	–	–	–	–	–	–	–
120 cm	1.30	0.97	1.38	1.07	1.40	1.11	1.41	1.13	–	–	–	–	–	–	–	–
125 cm	1.43	1.07	1.52	1.18	1.54	1.22	1.55	1.24	–	–	–	–	–	–	–	–
130 cm	1.57	1.17	1.66	1.29	1.69	1.34	1.70	1.36	1.74	1.41	–	–	–	–	–	–
135 cm	–	–	–	–	1.85	1.46	1.85	1.49	1.90	1.54	–	–	–	–	–	–
140 cm	–	–	–	–	2.01	1.59	2.02	1.62	2.07	1.67	2.21	1.80	–	–	–	–
145 cm	–	–	–	–	2.18	1.73	2.19	1.76	2.24	1.82	2.40	1.95	2.60	2.12	2.75	2.24
150 cm	–	–	–	–	–	–	2.37	1.91	2.43	1.97	2.60	2.11	2.82	2.29	2.97	2.42
155 cm	–	–	–	–	–	–	2.56	2.06	2.62	2.12	2.81	2.28	3.04	2.48	3.21	2.62
160 cm	–	–	–	–	–	–	2.76	2.22	2.83	2.29	3.02	2.46	3.28	2.67	3.46	2.82
165 cm	–	–	–	–	–	–	–	–	3.04	2.46	3.25	2.64	3.52	2.87	3.72	3.03
170 cm	–	–	–	–	–	–	–	–	3.26	2.63	3.48	2.83	3.78	3.07	3.99	3.25
175 cm	–	–	–	–	–	–	–	–	–	–	3.73	3.03	4.04	3.29	4.27	3.48
180 cm	–	–	–	–	–	–	–	–	–	–	3.98	3.23	4.32	3.51	4.56	3.71
185 cm	–	–	–	–	–	–	–	–	–	–	4.25	3.45	4.60	3.75	4.86	3.96
190 cm	–	–	–	–	–	–	–	–	–	–	4.52	3.67	4.90	3.99	5.17	4.22
195 cm	–	–	–	–	–	–	–	–	–	–	–	–	5.20	4.24	5.50	4.48

Source: Stanojevic et al. (2009).

TABLE C.18 — Predicted normal values: mean and lower limit of normal FVC (L) MALE CHILDREN

Age (yrs)	4 Mean	4 LLN	6 Mean	6 LLN	8 Mean	8 LLN	10 Mean	10 LLN	12 Mean	12 LLN	14 Mean	14 LLN	16 Mean	16 LLN	18 Mean	18 LLN
110 cm	1.11	0.82	1.22	0.94	1.28	1.01	–	1.17	–	–	–	–	–	–	–	–
115 cm	1.24	0.92	1.36	1.04	1.42	1.12	1.46	1.30	–	–	–	–	–	–	–	–
120 cm	1.38	1.02	1.51	1.16	1.58	1.25	1.62	1.44	–	–	–	–	–	–	–	–
125 cm	1.52	1.12	1.66	1.28	1.74	1.38	1.79	1.58	2.01	1.64	–	–	–	–	–	–
130 cm	1.67	1.23	1.83	1.41	1.92	1.51	1.97	1.73	2.21	1.79	–	–	–	–	–	–
135 cm	–	–	–	–	2.10	1.66	2.15	1.89	2.41	1.96	2.57	2.10	–	–	–	–
140 cm	–	–	–	–	2.30	1.81	2.35	2.06	2.63	2.13	2.80	2.29	–	–	–	–
145 cm	–	–	–	–	2.50	1.98	2.56	2.24	2.85	2.32	3.04	2.49	3.04	2.50	3.22	2.66
150 cm	–	–	–	–	–	–	2.79	2.42	3.09	2.51	3.29	2.70	3.30	2.72	3.50	2.89
155 cm	–	–	–	–	–	–	3.02	2.62	3.34	2.71	3.56	2.91	3.58	2.94	3.79	3.13
160 cm	–	–	–	–	–	–	3.26	–	3.60	2.92	3.84	3.14	3.86	3.18	4.09	3.38
165 cm	–	–	–	–	–	–	–	–	3.87	3.15	4.13	3.38	4.17	3.43	4.41	3.64
170 cm	–	–	–	–	–	–	–	–	–	–	4.43	3.63	4.48	3.69	4.75	3.92
175 cm	–	–	–	–	–	–	–	–	–	–	4.74	3.88	4.81	3.96	5.09	4.20
180 cm	–	–	–	–	–	–	–	–	–	–	5.07	4.15	5.15	4.24	5.45	4.50
185 cm	–	–	–	–	–	–	–	–	–	–	5.41	4.43	5.50	4.53	5.83	4.81
190 cm	–	–	–	–	–	–	–	–	–	–	–	–	5.87	4.83	6.22	5.14
195 cm	–	–	–	–	–	–	–	–	–	–	–	–	6.26	5.15	6.63	5.47

Source: Stanojevic et al. (2009).

TABLE C.19 Predicted normal values: mean and lower limit of normal FEV$_1$/FVC MALE CHILDREN

Age (yrs)	4 Mean	4 LLN	6 Mean	6 LLN	8 Mean	8 LLN	10 Mean	10 LLN	12 Mean	12 LLN	14 Mean	14 LLN	16 Mean	16 LLN	18 Mean	18 LLN
110 cm	0.95	0.86	0.93	0.8	0.90	0.78	–	–	–	–	–	–	–	–	–	–
115 cm	0.95	0.85	0.92	0.8	0.90	0.78	0.88	0.75	–	–	–	–	–	–	–	–
120 cm	0.95	0.85	0.92	0.8	0.90	0.78	0.88	0.75	–	–	–	–	–	–	–	–
125 cm	0.95	0.85	0.92	0.8	0.89	0.78	0.87	0.75	–	–	–	–	–	–	–	–
130 cm	0.95	0.85	0.92	0.8	0.89	0.78	0.87	0.75	–	–	–	–	–	–	–	–
135 cm	–	–	–	–	0.89	0.78	0.87	0.75	0.87	0.74	–	–	–	–	–	–
140 cm	–	–	–	–	0.89	0.77	0.87	0.75	0.86	0.74	0.86	0.73	–	–	–	–
145 cm	–	–	–	–	0.89	0.77	0.87	0.75	0.86	0.74	0.86	0.73	0.86	0.73	0.86	0.72
150 cm	–	–	–	–	–	–	0.87	0.75	0.86	0.74	0.86	0.73	0.86	0.73	0.85	0.72
155 cm	–	–	–	–	–	–	0.87	0.75	0.86	0.74	0.86	0.73	0.86	0.72	0.85	0.72
160 cm	–	–	–	–	–	–	–	–	0.86	0.73	0.86	0.73	0.86	0.72	0.85	0.72
165 cm	–	–	–	–	–	–	–	–	0.86	0.73	0.86	0.73	0.86	0.72	0.85	0.72
170 cm	–	–	–	–	–	–	–	–	0.86	0.73	0.86	0.73	0.85	0.72	0.85	0.72
175 cm	–	–	–	–	–	–	–	–	0.86	0.73	0.86	0.73	0.85	0.72	0.85	0.72
180 cm	–	–	–	–	–	–	–	–	–	–	0.85	0.73	0.85	0.72	0.85	0.72
185 cm	–	–	–	–	–	–	–	–	–	–	0.85	0.72	0.85	0.72	0.85	0.72
190 cm	–	–	–	–	–	–	–	–	–	–	0.85	0.72	0.85	0.72	0.85	0.71
195 cm	–	–	–	–	–	–	–	–	–	–	–	–	0.85	0.72	0.85	0.71

Source: Stanojevic et al. (2009).

TABLE C.20 — Predicted normal values: mean and lower limit of normal FEF$_{25-75\%}$ (L/sec) MALE CHILDREN

Age (yrs)	4 Mean	4 LLN	6 Mean	6 LLN	8 Mean	8 LLN	10 Mean	10 LLN	12 Mean	12 LLN	14 Mean	14 LLN	16 Mean	16 LLN	18 Mean	18 LLN
110 cm	1.52	0.91	1.50	0.92	1.50	0.93	–	–	–	–	–	–	–	–	–	–
115 cm	1.65	0.99	1.63	1.00	1.62	1.01	1.65	1.05	–	–	–	–	–	–	–	–
120 cm	1.78	1.07	1.76	1.08	1.75	1.09	1.78	1.13	–	–	–	–	–	–	–	–
125 cm	1.91	1.15	1.90	1.16	1.89	1.18	1.92	1.22	2.17	1.39	–	–	–	–	–	–
130 cm	2.06	1.24	2.03	1.25	2.03	1.26	2.06	1.31	2.32	1.49	–	–	–	–	–	–
135 cm	–	–	–	–	2.17	1.35	2.21	1.40	2.48	1.59	–	–	–	–	–	–
140 cm	–	–	–	–	2.32	1.44	2.36	1.49	2.64	1.69	2.66	1.72	–	–	–	–
145 cm	–	–	–	–	2.47	1.54	2.51	1.59	2.80	1.80	2.84	1.83	3.04	1.98	3.18	2.08
150 cm	–	–	–	–	–	–	2.67	1.69	2.98	1.91	3.01	1.95	3.23	2.10	3.38	2.21
155 cm	–	–	–	–	–	–	2.83	1.79	3.15	2.02	3.20	2.07	3.43	2.23	3.59	2.34
160 cm	–	–	–	–	–	–	3.00	1.90	3.33	2.13	3.39	2.19	3.63	2.36	3.80	2.48
165 cm	–	–	–	–	–	–	–	–	3.52	2.25	3.58	2.31	3.84	2.50	4.02	2.62
170 cm	–	–	–	–	–	–	–	–	–	–	3.78	2.44	4.05	2.63	4.24	2.77
175 cm	–	–	–	–	–	–	–	–	–	–	3.98	2.57	4.27	2.78	4.47	2.92
180 cm	–	–	–	–	–	–	–	–	–	–	4.19	2.71	4.49	2.92	4.70	3.07
185 cm	–	–	–	–	–	–	–	–	–	–	4.40	2.85	4.72	3.07	4.94	3.22
190 cm	–	–	–	–	–	–	–	–	–	–	4.62	2.99	4.95	3.22	5.18	3.38
195 cm	–	–	–	–	–	–	–	–	–	–	–	–	5.19	3.37	5.43	3.55

Source: Stanojevic et al. (2009).

TABLE C.21	Predicted normal values: mean and lower limit of normal PEF (L/min) MALE CHILDREN												
Age (yrs)	8		10		12		14		16		18		20	
	Mean	LLN	Mean	LLN	Mean	LLN	Mean	LLN	Mean	LLN	Mean	LLN	Mean	LLN
130 cm	208	134	222	148	242	168	268	194	300	226	339	265	384	310
135 cm	228	148	242	162	262	182	288	208	320	240	359	279	404	324
140 cm	249	163	262	176	282	196	308	222	341	255	380	294	425	339
145 cm	270	178	284	191	304	211	330	237	362	270	401	309	446	354
150 cm	292	193	306	207	326	227	352	253	384	285	423	324	468	369
155 cm	315	210	329	223	349	243	375	269	407	302	446	340	491	385
160 cm	339	226	352	240	372	260	398	286	431	318	470	357	515	402
165 cm	363	243	377	257	396	277	423	303	455	335	494	374	539	419
170 cm	388	261	402	275	422	295	448	321	480	353	519	392	564	437
175 cm	414	279	428	293	447	313	474	339	506	371	545	410	590	455
180 cm	441	298	454	312	474	332	500	358	533	390	571	429	616	474
185 cm	468	317	481	331	501	351	527	377	560	409	599	448	644	493

Source: Hankinson, Odencrantz & Fedan (1999).

TABLE C.22 Predicted normal values: mean and lower limit of normal FEV$_1$ (L) FEMALE CHILDREN

Age (yrs)	4 Mean	4 LLN	6 Mean	6 LLN	8 Mean	8 LLN	10 Mean	10 LLN	12 Mean	12 LLN	14 Mean	14 LLN	16 Mean	16 LLN	18 Mean	18 LLN
110 cm	1.03	0.77	1.07	0.82	1.10	0.86	–	1.00	–	–	–	–	–	–	–	–
115 cm	1.14	0.85	1.18	0.91	1.22	0.95	1.27	1.10	–	–	–	–	–	–	–	–
120 cm	1.25	0.93	1.30	1.00	1.34	1.05	1.39	1.21	1.48	1.18	–	–	–	–	–	–
125 cm	1.37	1.02	1.42	1.09	1.46	1.14	1.53	1.32	1.62	1.29	–	–	–	–	–	–
130 cm	1.49	1.12	1.55	1.19	1.59	1.25	1.66	1.43	1.76	1.41	–	–	–	–	–	–
135 cm	–	–	–	–	1.73	1.36	1.81	1.55	1.91	1.53	2.19	1.76	–	–	–	–
140 cm	–	–	–	–	1.88	1.47	1.96	1.67	2.07	1.65	2.37	1.90	2.46	1.99	2.52	2.04
145 cm	–	–	–	–	2.03	1.59	2.11	1.80	2.24	1.79	2.55	2.05	2.66	2.14	2.71	2.19
150 cm	–	–	–	–	–	–	2.28	1.94	2.41	1.93	2.74	2.20	2.85	2.30	2.92	2.36
155 cm	–	–	–	–	–	–	2.45	2.08	2.59	2.07	2.94	2.36	3.06	2.47	3.13	2.53
160 cm	–	–	–	–	–	–	2.62	–	2.78	2.22	3.15	2.53	3.27	2.64	3.35	2.71
165 cm	–	–	–	–	–	–	–	–	2.97	2.37	3.36	2.70	3.50	2.82	3.57	2.89
170 cm	–	–	–	–	–	–	–	–	3.18	2.54	3.58	2.88	3.73	3.00	3.81	3.08
175 cm	–	–	–	–	–	–	–	–	–	–	3.81	3.06	3.96	3.20	4.05	3.27
180 cm	–	–	–	–	–	–	–	–	–	–	4.05	3.25	4.21	3.40	4.30	3.48
185 cm	–	–	–	–	–	–	–	–	–	–	4.29	3.45	4.47	3.60	4.56	3.69
190 cm	–	–	–	–	–	–	–	–	–	–	–	–	–	–	4.83	3.90
195 cm	–	–	–	–	–	–	–	–	–	–	–	–	–	–	–	–

Source: Stanojevic et al. (2009).

TABLE C.23 — Predicted normal values: mean and lower limit of normal FVC (L) FEMALE CHILDREN

Age (yrs)	4 Mean	4 LLN	6 Mean	6 LLN	8 Mean	8 LLN	10 Mean	10 LLN	12 Mean	12 LLN	14 Mean	14 LLN	16 Mean	16 LLN	18 Mean	18 LLN
110 cm	1.08	0.79	1.15	0.87	1.21	0.95	–	–	–	–	–	–	–	–	–	–
115 cm	1.19	0.87	1.28	0.97	1.34	1.05	1.40	1.12	–	–	–	–	–	–	–	–
120 cm	1.32	0.96	1.41	1.07	1.48	1.16	1.54	1.24	1.62	1.31	–	–	–	–	–	–
125 cm	1.45	1.06	1.55	1.18	1.63	1.28	1.70	1.36	1.78	1.45	–	–	–	–	–	–
130 cm	1.59	1.16	1.70	1.29	1.78	1.40	1.86	1.49	1.95	1.59	–	–	–	–	–	–
135 cm	–	–	–	–	1.95	1.53	2.03	1.63	2.13	1.73	–	–	–	–	–	–
140 cm	–	–	–	–	2.12	1.66	2.21	1.77	2.32	1.89	2.44	2.00	–	–	–	–
145 cm	–	–	–	–	2.30	1.80	2.40	1.92	2.52	2.05	2.65	2.17	2.76	2.27	2.83	2.33
150 cm	–	–	–	–	–	–	2.60	2.08	2.73	2.21	2.87	2.35	2.98	2.45	3.06	2.52
155 cm	–	–	–	–	–	–	2.80	2.25	2.94	2.39	3.10	2.53	3.22	2.65	3.30	2.72
160 cm	–	–	–	–	–	–	3.02	2.42	3.17	2.57	3.33	2.73	3.47	2.85	3.56	2.93
165 cm	–	–	–	–	–	–	–	–	3.41	2.77	3.58	2.93	3.73	3.06	3.82	3.15
170 cm	–	–	–	–	–	–	–	–	3.65	2.97	3.84	3.14	4.00	3.28	4.10	3.38
175 cm	–	–	–	–	–	–	–	–	–	–	4.11	3.36	4.28	3.51	4.39	3.62
180 cm	–	–	–	–	–	–	–	–	–	–	4.39	3.59	4.28	3.51	4.68	3.86
185 cm	–	–	–	–	–	–	–	–	–	–	4.68	3.83	4.57	3.75	4.99	4.11
190 cm	–	–	–	–	–	–	–	–	–	–	4.98	4.07	4.87	4.00	5.31	4.38
195 cm	–	–	–	–	–	–	–	–	–	–	–	–	5.18	4.26	5.65	4.65

Source: Stanojevic et al. (2009).

TABLE C.24 Predicted normal values: mean and lower limit of normal FEV₁/FVC FEMALE CHILDREN

Age (yrs)	4		6		8		10		12		14		16		18	
	Mean	LLN	Mean	LLN	Mean	LLN	Mean	LLN	Mean	LLN	Mean	LLN	Mean	LLN	Mean	LLN
110 cm	0.96	0.87	0.94	0.83	0.96	0.92	–	–	–	–	–	–	–	–	–	–
115 cm	0.95	0.86	0.93	0.83	0.91	0.80	0.91	0.79	–	–	–	–	–	–	–	–
120 cm	0.95	0.86	0.93	0.83	0.91	0.80	0.90	0.79	0.91	0.79	–	–	–	–	–	–
125 cm	0.95	0.86	0.93	0.82	0.91	0.80	0.90	0.78	0.90	0.78	–	–	–	–	–	–
130 cm	0.94	0.85	0.92	0.82	0.91	0.79	0.90	0.78	0.90	0.78	–	–	–	–	–	–
135 cm	–	–	–	–	0.90	0.79	0.90	0.78	0.90	0.78	–	–	–	–	–	–
140 cm	–	–	–	–	0.90	0.79	0.89	0.78	0.90	0.78	0.90	0.78	0.90	0.78	–	–
145 cm	–	–	–	–	0.90	0.79	0.89	0.77	0.89	0.77	0.90	0.78	0.90	0.77	0.90	0.77
150 cm	–	–	–	–	–	–	0.89	0.77	0.89	0.77	0.90	0.77	0.89	0.77	0.90	0.77
155 cm	–	–	–	–	–	–	0.89	0.77	0.89	0.77	0.89	0.77	0.89	0.77	0.89	0.77
160 cm	–	–	–	–	–	–	0.88	–	0.89	0.77	0.89	0.77	0.89	0.77	0.89	0.77
165 cm	–	–	–	–	–	–	–	–	0.88	0.77	0.89	0.77	0.89	0.77	0.89	0.76
170 cm	–	–	–	–	–	–	–	–	0.88	0.77	0.89	0.77	0.88	0.76	0.88	0.76
175 cm	–	–	–	–	–	–	–	–	–	–	0.88	0.77	0.88	0.76	0.88	0.76
180 cm	–	–	–	–	–	–	–	–	–	–	0.88	0.76	0.88	0.76	0.88	0.76
185 cm	–	–	–	–	–	–	–	–	–	–	0.88	0.76	0.88	0.76	0.88	0.76
190 cm	–	–	–	–	–	–	–	–	–	–	0.88	0.76	0.88	0.76	0.88	0.76
195 cm	–	–	–	–	–	–	–	–	–	–	–	–	–	–	0.87	0.75

Source: Stanojevic et al. (2009).

TABLE C.25 — Predicted normal values: mean and lower limit of normal FEF$_{25-75\%}$ (L/sec) FEMALE CHILDREN

Age (yrs)	4 Mean	4 LLN	6 Mean	6 LLN	8 Mean	8 LLN	10 Mean	10 LLN	12 Mean	12 LLN	14 Mean	14 LLN	16 Mean	16 LLN	18 Mean	18 LLN
110 cm	1.49	0.91	1.51	0.95	1.57	1.01	–	–	–	–	–	–	–	–	–	–
115 cm	1.60	0.98	1.62	1.02	1.68	1.08	–	–	–	–	–	–	–	–	–	–
120 cm	1.71	1.05	1.73	1.09	1.80	1.16	1.80	1.17	–	–	–	–	–	–	–	–
125 cm	1.83	1.12	1.85	1.17	1.93	1.24	1.93	1.26	2.06	1.36	–	–	–	–	–	–
130 cm	1.95	1.20	1.97	1.25	2.05	1.32	2.06	1.34	2.20	1.45	–	–	–	–	–	–
135 cm	–	–	–	–	2.18	1.41	2.19	1.43	2.35	1.55	–	–	–	–	–	–
140 cm	–	–	–	–	2.31	1.49	2.33	1.52	2.50	1.64	2.80	1.85	–	–	–	–
145 cm	–	–	–	–	2.45	1.58	2.47	1.61	2.65	1.74	2.96	1.95	–	–	3.11	2.06
150 cm	–	–	–	–	–	–	2.62	1.71	2.80	1.84	3.12	2.06	3.06	2.02	3.29	2.17
155 cm	–	–	–	–	–	–	2.76	1.80	2.96	1.95	3.29	2.18	3.23	2.14	3.47	2.25
160 cm	–	–	–	–	–	–	2.91	1.90	3.12	2.05	3.47	2.29	3.41	2.25	3.65	2.41
165 cm	–	–	–	–	–	–	3.07	2.00	3.28	2.16	3.64	2.41	3.59	2.37	3.83	2.53
170 cm	–	–	–	–	–	–	–	–	3.45	2.27	3.82	2.53	3.77	2.49	4.02	2.66
175 cm	–	–	–	–	–	–	–	–	3.62	2.38	4.01	2.65	3.96	2.62	4.22	2.78
180 cm	–	–	–	–	–	–	–	–	–	–	4.19	2.77	4.15	2.74	4.41	2.90
185 cm	–	–	–	–	–	–	–	–	–	–	4.38	2.89	4.34	2.87	4.61	3.04
190 cm	–	–	–	–	–	–	–	–	–	–	4.58	3.02	4.53	3.00	4.81	3.17
195 cm	–	–	–	–	–	–	–	–	–	–	–	–	4.73	3.13	5.02	3.31

Source: Stanojevic et al. (2009).

TABLE C.26	Predicted normal values: mean and lower limit of normal PEF (L/min) FEMALE CHILDREN											
Age (yrs)	8		10		12		14		16		18	
	Mean	LLN	Mean	LLN	Mean	LLN	Mean	LLN	Mean	LLN	Mean	LLN
120 cm	170	114	207	151	235	179	255	199	267	211	271	215
125 cm	184	123	220	160	249	188	269	208	281	220	285	224
130 cm	198	132	235	169	263	197	283	217	295	230	299	234
135 cm	213	142	249	179	278	207	298	227	310	239	314	243
140 cm	228	152	265	189	293	217	313	237	325	249	329	253
145 cm	244	163	281	199	309	227	329	247	341	260	345	264
150 cm	261	173	297	210	325	238	346	258	358	270	362	274
155 cm	278	184	314	221	342	249	363	269	375	281	379	285
160 cm	295	196	332	232	360	261	380	281	392	293	396	297
165 cm	314	208	350	244	378	272	398	293	411	305	415	309
170 cm	332	220	369	256	397	285	417	305	429	317	433	321
175 cm	352	233	388	269	416	297	436	317	449	330	453	334
180 cm	371	245	408	282	436	310	456	330	468	342	472	347
185 cm	392	259	428	295	456	323	477	344	489	356	493	360

Source: Hankinson, Odencrantz & Fedan (1999).

ANZSRS	Australian and New Zealand Society of Respiratory Science (www.anzsrs.org.au)
ARTP	Association of Respiratory Technology and Physiology (www.artp.org.uk)
ATPS	Ambient temperature and pressure saturated with water vapour.
ATS	American Thoracic Society (www.thoracic.org)
Back-extrapolation	Procedure applied to the maximal expiratory spirogram (volume versus time) to determine zero time. The zero time point is the point on the time axis where exhalation would have started, assuming 'instantaneous' flow acceleration (the patient's maximal flow is projected back to the volume axis) and is used for the calculation of FEV_1.
BTPS	Body temperature (37°C) and pressure saturated with water vapour (47 mmHg). All volumes and flows are reported after conversion to BTPS conditions.
ERS	European Respiratory Society (www.ersnet.org)
$FEF_{25-75\%}$	Forced expiratory flow over the middle half of the FVC manoeuvre. This is the average expired flow over the middle half of the FVC manoeuvre. Normally reported in L/s. In Europe this is often referred to as the $MEF_{25-75\%}$ or MMEF (maximum mid-expiratory flow).

FEF$_{25-75\%6}$ Forced expiratory flow over the middle half of the FVC$_6$ manoeuvre. Normally reported in L/s.

FEF$_{50\%}$ Forced expiratory flow at 50% of the FVC. This is the maximal expiratory flow measured at the point where 50% of the FVC has been expired. Normally reported in L/s. In Europe this is often referred to as the MEF$_{50\%}$.

FEF$_{75\%}$ Forced expiratory flow at 75% FVC. This is the maximal expiratory flow measured at the point where 75% has been expired. Normally reported in L/s. In Europe this is often referred to as the MEF$_{25\%}$.

FET   Forced expiratory time. This is the time (in seconds) required to perform the FVC manoeuvre.

FEV$_1$ Forced expired volume in 1 second. This is the volume expired (in L or mL) in the first second of maximal expiration (initiated after a maximal inspiration).

FEV$_1$/FVC ratio (FEV$_1$/VC)   The FEV$_1$ expressed as a fraction of the FVC (or VC). The normal ratio is usually within the range 0.75 to 0.85, but is age-dependent. Lung disease can increase or decrease the ratio. This is also referred to as the forced expiratory ratio, FER.

FEV$_6$ Similar to FVC$_6$ (see below) but is the forced expired volume measured *at* 6 seconds.

FEV$_1$/FVC$_6$ ratio   FEV$_1$ expressed as a fraction of the FVC$_6$. Lung disease can increase or decrease this ratio.

FIV$_1$ Forced inspired volume in 1 second (L or mL). Maximum volume that can be inspired from residual volume in 1 second.

FIVC   Forced inspired vital capacity (L or mL). Maximum volume that can be inspired from residual volume.

Flow-volume loop   A plot of maximal expired and inspired volume versus flow. Most of the expiratory curve is effort-independent and the entire inspiratory curve is effort-dependent.

FRC	Function residual capacity (L or mL), that is, the resting volume of the lungs.
FVC	Forced vital capacity (L or mL). The maximum volume of air that can be expired or inspired during a forced expiratory manoeuvre initiated from TLC or RV.
FVC$_6$	Largest forced expiratory volume (L or mL) measured during the first 6 seconds.
Hyperinflation	This term refers to a significant increase in static lung volumes—total lung capacity or functional residual capacity. Dynamic increase in functional residual capacity can occur particularly in subjects with airflow obstruction when expiratory time is insufficient, for instance when breathing rate is increased during exercise.
Inspiratory capacity (IC)	The maximum volume of air that can be inspired from functional residual capacity. Normally reported in L or mL.
Kymograph	Rotating drum used with manual displacement spirometers to record time and respired volume.
Mannitol	Indirect bronchial provocation agent used to identify bronchial hyperresponsiveness in people suspected of having asthma.
Methacholine	Non-specific bronchial agent that can induce airway constriction. The dose of methacholine that induces a 20% decrease in FEV$_1$ from the control value is referred to as the PD$_{20\%}$.
Mixed ventilatory defect	Characterised by *both* airflow limitation (obstruction) and loss of lung volume (lung restriction). Produces both a low FEV$_1$/FVC ratio and low VC (or FVC). The restrictive component should be confirmed and quantified by formal measurement of lung volume (for example, multi-breath inert gas dilution, nitrogen washout or whole body plethysmography).
NAC	National Asthma Council of Australia (www.nationalasthma.org.au)

Obstructive ventilatory defect	Characterised by airflow limitation, for example, reduced FEV_1, FEV_1/FVC ratio or PEF. The term 'airflow limitation' is also used and is, perhaps, a more accurate term than 'obstruction' as reduced expired flows can arise not only due to abnormal airway calibre, but also in altered parenchymal compliance and impaired mechanical linkage between airways and lung parenchyma.
P_b	Barometric pressure (mmHg).
$PD_{20\%}$	Dose of provoking agent (e.g. methacholine) required to decrease the FEV_1 (or PEF) by 20% from the baseline value.
PEF	Peak expiratory flow (L/s or L/min). This is the maximal expiratory flow achieved during a maximum forced expiration initiated at TLC. The PEF is effort-dependent and occurs very early in the forced expiratory manoeuvre.
PIF	Peak inspiratory flow (L/s or L/min). This is the maximal inspiratory flow achieved during a maximum forced inspiration initiated at residual volume.
Pneumotachograph	Device for measuring flow from the pressure drop across a uniform and known resistance under conditions of laminar flow.
Restrictive ventilatory defect	Characterised by loss of lung volume in the absence of airflow limitation, as suggested by a low VC or FVC but normal or high FEV_1/FVC ratio. If lung restriction is suspected on spirometry, formal measurements of lung volumes should be done to confirm and quantify it (e.g. multi-breath inert gas dilution, nitrogen washout or whole body plethysmography).
Reversibility	Improvement in ventilatory function (for instance, FEV_1) following the inhalation of a bronchodilator:

$$\% \text{ improvement} = 100 \times \frac{FEV_1 \text{ (post–bronchodilator)} - FEV_1 \text{ (baseline)}}{FEV_1 \text{ (baseline)}}$$

Significant reversibility is implied if there is a $\geq 12\%$ improvement in FEV_1 (or FVC) *and* an absolute improvement of ≥ 0.2 L.

Spirogram   A plot of respired volume versus time.

Spirometer   Device used to measure respired volume. Spirometers may be classified as either volume or flow spirometers depending on whether the primary signal measured is volume or flow.

Spirometry   Physiological test to measure the ventilatory function of the lungs.

TLC   Total lung capacity (L or mL). Total volume contained within the lung at full inspiration.

TSANZ   Thoracic Society of Australia and New Zealand (www.thoracic.org.au)

VC   Vital capacity (L or mL). The maximum volume of air that can be expired or inspired during a slow manoeuvre initiated at TLC or residual volume, respectively.

Bracci M, Strafella E, Croce N, Staffolani S, Carducci A, Verani M, Valentino M & Santarelli L 2011, 'Risk of bacterial cross infection associated with inspiration through flow-based spirometers', *American Journal of Infection Control*, vol. 39, no. 1, pp. 50–5.

Burton D, Johns DP & Swanney M 2011, *Spirometer Users' and Buyers' Guide*, Australian Government Department of Health and Ageing, Canberra, www.nationalasthma.org.au.

Crapo RO 1994, 'Pulmonary function testing', *New England Journal of Medicine*, vol. 331, pp. 25–30.

Enright PL, Connett JE & Bailey WC 2002, 'The FEV1/FEV6 predicts lung function decline in adult smokers', *Respiratory Medicine*, vol. 96, no. 6, pp. 444–9.

Fardy HJ 2001, 'Spirometry: Value adding in GP asthma care', *GP Review* (Asthma update), September, vol. 5, no. 9, p. 21.

Ferguson GT, Enright PL, Buist AS & Higgins MW 2000, 'Office spirometry for health assessment in adults: a consensus statement from the National Lung Health Education Program, *Chest*, vol. 117, pp. 1146–61.

Hancox B & Whyte K 2006, *McGraw-Hill's Pocket Guide to Lung Function Tests* (2nd edn), McGraw-Hill, Sydney.

Hankinson JL, Odencrantz JR & Fedan KB 1999, 'Spirometric reference values from a sample of the general US population', *American Journal of Respiratory and Critical Care Medicine*, vol. 159, pp. 179–87.

Hankinson JL, Crapo RO & Jensen RL 2003, 'Spirometric reference values for the 6-s FVC maneuver', *Chest*, vol. 124, pp. 1805–11.

Jacques I, Derelle J, Weber M & Vidailhet M 1998, 'Pulmonary evolution of cystic fibrosis patients colonized by Pseudomonas aeruginosa and/or Burkholderia cepacia', *European Journal of Pediatrics*, vol. 157, no. 5, pp. 427–31.

Johns DP, Ingram C, Booth H, Williams TJ & Walters EH 1995, 'Effect of micro-aerosol filter on the measurement of lung function', *Chest*, vol. 107, pp. 1045–8.

Johns DP, Hartley MF, Burns G & Thompson BR 2004, 'Variation in barometric pressure in Melbourne does not significantly affect the BTPS correction factor', *Respirology*, vol. 9, pp. 406–8.

Kendrick AH, Johns DP & Leeming JP 2003, 'Infection control of lung function equipment: a practical approach', *Respiratory Medicine*, vol. 97, no. 11, pp. 1163–79.

Miller MR, Crapo R, Hankinson J, Brusasco V, Burgos F, Casaburi R, Coates A, Enright P, van der Grinten CPM, Gustafsson P, Jensen R, Johnson DC, MacIntyre N, McKay R, Navajas D, Pedersen OF, Pellegrino R, Viegi G & Wanger J 2005a, 'General considerations for lung function testing', *European Respiratory Journal*, vol. 26, no. 1, pp. 153–62.

Miller MR, Hankinson J, Brusasco V, Burgos F, Casaburi R, Coates A, Crapo RO, Enright P, van der Grinten CPM, Gustafsson P, Jensen R, Johnson DC, MacIntyre N, McKay R, Navajas D, Pedersen OF, Pellegrino R, Viegi G & Wanger J 2005b, 'Standardisation of spirometry', *European Respiratory Journal*, vol. 26, pp. 319–38.

National Asthma Council (NAC) Australia 2006, *Asthma Management Handbook*, NAC, Melbourne.

O'Donnell DE 2000, 'Assessment of bronchodilator efficacy in symptomatic COPD', *Chest*, vol. 117, no. 2, pp. S425–S75.

Pellegrino R, Viegi G, Brusasco V, Crapo RO, Burgos F, Casaburi R, Coates A, van der Grinten CPM, Gustafsson P, Hankinson J, Jensen R, Johnson DC, MacIntyre N, McKay R, Miller MR, Navajas D, Pedersen OF & Wanger J 2005, 'Interpretative strategies for lung function tests', *European Respiratory Journal*, vol. 26, pp. 948–68.

Pierce R & Johns DP 1995, *Spirometry: The Measurement and Interpretation of Ventilatory Function in Clinical Practice*, National Asthma Campaign, Melbourne, viewed 21 March 2011, www.nationalasthma.org.au.

Quanjer PH, Tammeling GJ, Cotes JE, Petersen OF, Peslin R & Yernault JC 1993, 'Lung volumes and forced ventilatory flows. Report Working Party Standardization of Lung Function Tests, European Community for Steel and Coal. Official Statement of the European Respiratory Society', *European Respiratory Society*, vol. 6 (Suppl. 16), pp. 4–40.

Side EA, Harrington G, Thien F, Walters EH & Johns DP 1999, 'A cost-analysis of two approaches to infection control in a lung function laboratory', *Australian and New Zealand Journal of Medicine*, vol. 29, pp. 9–14.

Skloot GS, Edwards NT & Enright PL 2010, 'Four-year calibration of the EasyOne portable spirometer', *Respiratory Care*, vol. 55, no. 7, pp. 873–7.

Stanojevic S, Wade A, Cole TJ, Lum S, Custovic A, Silverman M, Hall GL, Welsh L, Kirby J, Nystad W, Badier M, Davis S, Turner S, Piccioni P, Vilozni D, Eigen H, Vlachos-Mayer H, Zheng J, Tomalak W, Jones M, Hankinson JL, Stocks J & Asthma UK Spirometry Collaborative Group 2009, 'Spirometry centile charts for young Caucasian children: the Asthma UK Collaborative Initiative', *American Journal of Respiratory and Critical Care Medicine*, vol. 180, no. 6, pp. 547–52.

Swanney MP, Jensen RL, Crichton DA, Beckert LE, Cardno LA & Crapo RO 2000, 'FEV_6 is an acceptable surrogate for FVC in the spirometric diagnosis of airway obstruction and restriction', *American Journal of Respiratory Critical Care Medicine*, vol. 162, pp. 917–19.

Unstead M, Stearn MD, Cramer D, Chadwick MV & Wilson R 2006, 'An audit into the efficacy of single use bacterial/viral filters for the prevention of equipment contamination during lung function assessment', *Respiratory Medicine*, vol. 100, pp. 946–50.

Walters JAE, Wood-Baker R, Walls J & Johns DP 2006, 'Stability of the EasyOne ultrasonic spirometer for use in general practice', *Respirology*, vol. 11, no. 3, pp. 306–10.

USEFUL WEBSITES

American Association for Respiratory Care: www.aarc.org
American College of Chest Physicians (ACCP): www.chestnet.org
American Lung Association: www.lungusa.org
American Thoracic Society: www.thoracic.org
Asian Pacific Society of Respirology: www.apsresp.org
Association for Respiratory Technology & Physiology: www.artp.org.uk
Australian & New Zealand Society of Respiratory Science:
    www.anzsrs.org.au
The Australian Lung Foundation: www.lungfoundation.com.au
The British Thoracic Society: www.brit-thoracic.org.uk
The Canadian Society of Respiratory Therapists: www.csrt.com
The Canadian Thoracic Society: www.lung.ca/cts
European Respiratory Society: www.ersnet.org
National Asthma Council Australia (NAC):
    www.nationalasthma.org.au
National Health and Medical Research Council (NHMRC):
    www.nhmrc.gov.au
National Heart, Lung and Blood Institute (NHLBI):
    www.nhlbi.nih.gov
The National Institute for Occupational Safety and Health
    (NIOSH): http://www.cdc.gov/niosh
National Lung Health Education Program (NLHEP):
    www.nlhep.org/spirom1.html
NAC Spirometry Resources—Spirometer Users' and Buyers' Guide:
    http://www.nationalasthma.org.au/content/view/254/414
SpiroXpert (Become an expert in spirometry): www.spirxpert.com
The Thoracic Society of Australia & New Zealand (TSANZ):
    www.thoracic.org.au
World Health Organization (WHO): www.who.int/en

References to figures and tables are in *italics*.
References to terms in the glossary are followed by a 'g'.

3 litre calibration syringe, 17–18, *18*
6-second forced expiration, 7, 10

acceptability criteria, 26–7, *27–8*, 44
age, predicted values and, 39
airflow, 84–7, *85*, *see also* flow-volume
    loops; PEF; PIF
    corrected to BTPS, *99*, 99–102, *101*
    effect of pulmonary disease on, 93
    patterns of, 85–7, *86*
    production of, 84–5, *85*
airflow limitation (obstruction), 47–50,
    48, *49*, *52*, 52, *see also* obstructive
    ventilatory defects
    maximal airflow limitation, 87–9,
      88, *89*
    reversibility, 54–5
    theories of, 90–3
airway reactivity, *see*
    hyperresponsiveness
airways, *90*, 90–4
    provocation testing, 55–7
    resistance, 87, 91–3
ambient temperature and pressure
    (ATPS), *99*, 99–101, 129g
American Thoracic Society, 96, 98
ANZSRS (Australian and New
    Zealand Society of Respiratory
    Science), 129g
ARTP (Association of Respiratory
    Technology and Physiology), 129g

asthma, *49–50*, *52*, 93, *see also*
    bronchodilator reversibility
    case histories, 64–5, 70–1
    peak flow monitoring, 16, 57–9, *58*
    provocation testing, 55–7, *56*
    right tests for, 59–60
atmospheric temperature and
    pressure, *see* ATPS
ATPS (ambient temperature and
    pressure), *99*, 99–101, 129g
ATS (American Thoracic Society),
    129g

back-extrapolation, 28, *29*, 30, 129g
barometric pressure, 132g, *see also*
    BTPS
biological controls, 19–20, *20*
body temperature and pressure
    saturated with water, 12, 20–1,
    99, 99–101, *101*, 129g
body weight, predicted values and, 40
breathing, 84–94
breathing circuits, *see* closed-circuit
    spirometry; open-circuit
    spirometry
bronchi, 56–7, 80–1, 85–6
bronchioles, 85, *86*
bronchodilator reversibility, 35, *52*,
    54–5, 133g
BTPS, 12, 20–1, *99*, 99–101, *101*, 129g

calibration, 17–21, *18*, 34
carcinomas, *49*, 50, 76–7, 80–1
case histories, 61–83
    of normal function, 62–3
changes over time, *see* serial
    measurements
children, 16–17, 26, 58
    predicted normal values, *119–28*
chronic obstructive pulmonary
    disease, *45*, 45, *51*, 52, *53*
    case histories, 66–7
    right test for, 59–60
classification of abnormal ventilatory
    function, *45*, 45–53, *46*, *48–9*,
    51–3, *see also* case histories
clinical practice, xii, 21–2, 27, 34–5,
    see also patients
closed-circuit spirometry, 10, 23, *24*, 25–6
complications, 4–5
contamination, 36–8
contraindications, 4–5
controls, biological, 19–20, *20*
COPD, *45*, 45, *51*, 52, *53*
    case histories, 66–7
    right test for, 59–60
correction to BTPS, *see* BTPS
cough, *30–1*, 32, 82
cross-infection, 36–8

disposable equipment, 37–8
DLCO (diffusing capacity of the lung
    for carbon monoxide), 59
doctors' surgeries, viii, 21–2, 27, 34–5,
    see also patients

effort-dependent respiration, 87–9, *88*,
    89, 91–3
effort needed in spirometry, 25–6,
    30–1, 36–8, *89*, 93, *see also* pleural
    pressure
    case histories, 82
elastic recoil pressure, 91
emphysema, *49–50*, 93
equal pressure points (EPP), 90–1
equipment standards, 17, *96*, *97*, 98
ERS (European Respiratory Society),
    96, 98, 129g
ethnic origin, predicted values and,
    39–40
European Respiratory Society (ERS),
    96, 98, 129g
exercise tolerance, 50, 52
expiratory flow, 47, *49–50*, 52, 85, 87–9,

    88, *89*, 93, *see also* FEF;
    flow-volume loops
expiratory spirometry, 38, *46*, 48
    performance problems, *30*
extrapolation, *see* back-extrapolation

$FEF_{25-75\%}$ (forced expiratory flow at
    25-75% FVC), 7–8, *8*, 10, 44, 47–8,
    129–30g
    predicted normal values, 39, 102,
    106, *110*, *114*, *118*, *122*, *127*
$FEF_{25-75\%6}$ (forced expiratory flow at
    25-75% FVC_6), 130g
$FEF_{50\%}$ (forced expiratory flow at 50%
    FVC), 10–11, *11*, 130g
$FEF_{75\%}$ (forced expiratory flow at 75%
    FVC), 10–11, *11*, 130g
females, predicted normal values,
    111–18, *124–8*
FET (forced expiratory time), 7, *8*, 130g
FEV_1 (forced expired volume in 1
    second), 6, *8*, 44–5, *45*, 47, 52,
    59–60, 130g
    back-extrapolation, 28, *29*
    bronchodilator reversibility, 54–5
    predicted normal values, 39, *42*,
    102, *104*, *112*, *119*, *124*
    provocation testing, *56*, 56–7
FEV_1/FVC ratio, 6–7, 47–9, *48*, 52, 59,
    130g
    abnormal ventilatory function, *48*
    expressed as a fraction, xii
    instrument-related problems, 34
    predicted normal values, 39, *43*,
    102, *105*, *113*, *117*, *121*, *126*
FEV_1/FVC_6 ratio, 7, 10, 130g
    predicted normal values, 102, *109*
FEV_1/VC ratio, 7, 130g
FEV_6 (forced expiratory volume at
    6 seconds), 7, 130g
fibrosing alveolitis, 72–3
filters, 37–8
FIV_1, 130g
FIVC, 130g
flow, *see* airflow
flow-limiting segment, 91–2
flow spirometers, 10–12, *13*, 14–16,
    18, 34
    calibration, 17–18
    validation procedures, 98
flow-volume loops, *11*, 93, 130g
    abnormal ventilatory function,
    46, *49*, *51–2*, *53*

case histories, *62, 64, 66, 68, 72, 74, 76, 78, 80*
choosing the right test, 59
exercise tolerance and, *50, 52*
open and closed circuit, *24*
performance problems, *31*
forced expiratory flow, *see* FEF
forced expiratory time, *see* FET
forced expired volume, *see* FEV
forced respiratory manoeuvres, 85, *86, 88*
FRC (functional residual capacity), 50, 52, 131g
FVC (forced vital capacity), 6–7, *8*, 10, *45*, 47–9, *48*, 52, 59–60, 131g, *see also* FEV$_1$/FVC ratio
    abnormal ventilatory function, *48*
    back-extrapolation, 28, 30
    bronchodilator reversibility, 54–5
    classifying abnormal, *51–3*
    instrument-related problems, 34
    predicted normal values, 39, 102, *103, 111, 120, 125*
    reduced use of, 7, 10
FVC$_6$ (forced expiratory volume measured during the first 6 seconds), 7, 10, 131g
    predicted normal values, 102, *108, 116*

gas flow, 84–5, *85, see also* airflow
gender, predicted normal values and, 39, *42, 43, 103–28*
glossary, 129–3g
grading severity of defects, 53, *54*

height, predicted values and, 39
hyperinflation, *9*, 10, 47, 50, 52, *53*, 60, 131g
hyperresponsiveness, 55–7, *56*, 59

IC, *see* inspiratory capacity
indications for spirometry, 3–4
infection control, 36–8
inspiratory capacity (IC), *9*, 10, 24, 50, 52, *53*, 60, 131g
    case histories, 74–5
inspiratory flow, 50, 52, *53*, 85, *89*, 93, *see also* flow-volume loops; maximal inspiratory flow
    case histories, 75, 77, 79, 80–1
instrument-related problems, 34
interpretation of spirometry, 44–60

intra-thoracic forces, *90*
isovolume pressure-flow curves, 87, *88*

kymographs, 18–19, 34, 131g

laminar (streamlined) flow, 86, *86*
larynx, 50, 78–9, 88–9, 93
leaks, 18–19, 34
linearity, 17–18, *18*, 34
LLN (lower limit of normal), *42, 43*, 61, 102, *103–28*
lung function, 1–3, *2*,
    see also ventilatory function
    infection and, 36–7
    tests, 1–3, 36–7
lung volume, 47, 49–50, 52, 87–8, *88*,
    see also flow-volume loops; restrictive ventilatory defects

males, predicted normal values, *103–10, 119–23*
mannitol, 131g
maximal airflow limitation, 87–9, *88*
maximal expiratory flow (V$_{max}$), 50, 88–9, 91–3, *see also* FEF; PEF
    case histories, 79
maximal inspiratory flow, 10–11, 88–9, *89*, 93, *see also* PIF
maximal mid-expiratory flow rate, 7, *see also* FEF$_{25-75\%}$
mean predicted normal values, *see* predicted normal values
measurement devices, *see* monitoring devices; spirometers
methacholine, 56, 131g
mixed ventilatory defects, *45, 46*, 47, *48, 49*, 131–2g
    choosing the right test, 59–60
MMEFR, 7, *see also* FEF$_{25-75\%}$
monitoring devices, 16–17,
    see also peak flow meters
mouthpieces, 32, *33*, 34, 37–8
muscular dystrophy, 74–5

NAC (National Asthma Council of Australia), 131g
normal reference values, *see* predicted normal values
normal subjects
    biological controls, 19–20, *20*
    pre-employment tests, 62–3
nose clips, 24–5
nurses, 35

obstructive ventilatory defects, 3, *45*, *46*, 47–50, *48*, *49*, *51*, *52*, 132g, *see also* airflow limitation; asthma; COPD; small airways disease
case histories, 64–5, 66–7, 76–7, 78–9, 80–1
choosing the right test, 59–60
severity grading, *54*
occlusion (obstruction), *31*, 32, *33*
occupational assessment, 57, 57–9, 62–3, 95
open-circuit spirometry, 10, 23–4, *24*, 26

patients, *see also* case histories; normal subjects
performance issues, 23–6, *30–1*, 30–4, *33*, 93
self-monitoring, 16–17, 57, 57–9
patterns of airflow, 85–7
P_b (barometric pressure), 132g
$PD_{20\%}$ (provoking dose), 56, *56*, 132g
peak flow meters, 16–17, 21, 57, 57–9, *58*
case histories, 70–1
PEF (peak expiratory flow), *11*, 11, 26, 47, 87, 132g, *see also* airflow
case histories, 70–1
predicted normal values, 39, 102, *107*, *115*, *123*, *128*
self-monitoring, 16–17, 57, 57–9, *58*
performance problems, 23–6, *30–1*, 30–4, *33*, 93
pharynx, 88–9
PIF (peak inspiratory flow), *11*, 11, 132g
pleural pressure, 87–8, *88–9*, *90*, 90–1, *see also* effort needed in spirometry
pneumotachographs, *13*, 15, 37, 100, 132g
predicted normal values, 16–17, 39–41, *42*, *43*, 102, *103–28*, *see also* LLN (lower limit of normal)
preoperative risk assessment, 59, 68–9
pressure, *see* equal pressure points; pleural pressure
pressure-flow curves, 87, *88*
problems, *see* performance problems
provocation testing, 55–7
provoking dose ($PD_{20\%}$), *56*, 56, 132g
pulmonary disease, *see* respiratory disease
pulmonary fibrosis, 49–50

pulmonary function, *see* lung function

quality control, 17–21, *18*, *19*, 19, 34

recoil pressure, *90*, 90–3
reference values, *see* predicted normal values
repeatability criteria, 26–7, *27–8*
reporting, 26–7, *27–8*
respiratory disease
effect on airflow, 93
infection control, 36–7
right test for, 59–60
restrictive ventilatory defects, *45*, *46*, 47–9, *48*, *49*, *51*, *52*, 132–3g, *see also* FVC; VC
case histories, 72–3, 74–5
choosing the right test, 59–60
results, reporting of, 26–7, *27–8*
reversibility, *see* bronchodilator reversibility

screening, 62–3, 95
self-monitoring, 16–17, 57, 57–9
case histories, 70–1
sensors (pneumotachographs), *13*, 15, 37–8, 100, 132g
serial measurements, 44, *45*, 59–60
severity grading, 53, *54*
slow start (hesitation), *30–1*, 32, 82
small airways disease, 68–9, 93
smokers, 4, 7, 59, 93, 95
case histories, 64–5, 66–9, 76–7, 80–1, 82
spirograms, 6–7, *8–9*, 14–15, 133g, *see also* BTPS; performance problems
spirometers, *13*, 13–16, 133g, *see also* flow spirometers; volume-displacement spirometers
automatic calculations, 14–15
choice of, 21–2
infection control, 36–8
instrument-related problems with, 34
standards for, 97, *98*
spirometry, 23–35, 133g
acceptability criteria, 26–7, *27–8*, 44
case histories, 62–3, *82*, 82
changes over time, 44–5, *45*
choosing the right test, 59–60
indications for, 3–4
interpretation of, 44–60, *45*, *46*, *48–9*, *51–3*

performing, 23–6
training courses, xvii
standards, 96, 97, 98
streamlined flow, *86*, 86
syringes for calibration, 17–18, *18*

temperature, *see* BTPS
thorax, *90*
tidal breathing, 23, 25, 50, *52*–3, 85
time, spirometry changes over, *see*
        serial measurements
timing accuracy, 18–19
TLC, *see* total lung capacity
tongue occlusion, *31*, 32, *33*, 34
total lung capacity (TLC), *30*, 47, 49,
        52, *52*, *53*, 133g
trachea, *49*, 50, 76–7, 85–6, *86*
tracheomalacia, *49*
training in spirometry, xvii
transitional flow, *86*, 86
TSANZ (Thoracic Society of Australia
        and New Zealand), 133g
turbulent flow, *86*, 86–7

validation procedures, 98
VC (vital capacity), 6, 47, *48*, 87, *88*,
        133g, *see also* FEV$_1$/VC ratio;
        lung volume
ventilatory function, 2–3, *see also* lung
        function
    abnormal, *45*, 45–53, *46*, *48*–9, *51*–3
    case histories, 61–83
    interpretation of spirometry, 44–60
    measurement of, 6–12
    normal function, 62–3
    predicted normal values, 16–17,
            39–41, *42*, *43*, 102, *103*–28
vital capacity, *see* VC
V$_{max}$, *see* maximal expiratory flow
volume-displacement spirometers, 10,
        13, 14, 34
    calibration, 17–21
    validation procedures, 98

wave-speed theory, 92–3
websites, 137